"Forget *Sugar Busters*. Forget *The Zone*. If you want the real scoop on how carbohydrates and sugar affect your body, read this book by the world's leading researchers on the subject. It's the authoritative, last word on choosing foods to control your blood sugar."

—JEAN CARPER, best-selling author of
Miracle Cures, Stop Aging Now! and
Food—Your Miracle Medicine

■

"The Glucose Revolution is nutrition science for the 21st century. Clearly written, it gives the scientific rationale for why all carbohydrates are not created equal. It is a practical guide for both professionals and patients. The food suggestions and recipes are exciting and tasty."

—RICHARD N. PODELL, M.D., M.P.H.,
Clinical Professor, Department of Family Medicine,
UMDNJ–Robert Wood Johnson Medical School,
and co-author of *The G-Index Diet:
The Missing Link That Makes Permanent
Weight Loss Possible*

OTHER *GLUCOSE REVOLUTION* TITLES

The Glucose Revolution: The Authoritative Guide to the Glycemic Index—The Groundbreaking Medical Discovery

The Glucose Revolution Pocket Guide to Losing Weight

The Glucose Revolution Pocket Guide to the Top 100 Low Glycemic Foods

The Glucose Revolution Pocket Guide to Sports Nutrition

∎

FORTHCOMING:

The Glucose Revolution Pocket Guide to Sugar and Energy

The Glucose Revolution Pocket Guide to Your Heart

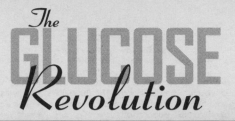

The GLUCOSE *Revolution*

POCKET GUIDE TO

DIABETES

KAYE FOSTER-POWELL, M. NUTR. & DIET.

JENNIE BRAND-MILLER, PH.D.

THOMAS M.S. WOLEVER, M.D., PH.D.

STEPHEN COLAGIURI, M.D.

ADAPTED BY

JOHANNA BURANI, M.S., R.D., C.D.E.

AND LINDA RAO, M.ED.

■

MARLOWE & COMPANY
NEW YORK

Published by
Marlowe & Company
841 Broadway, 4th Floor
New York, NY 10003

This book is not intended to replace the services of a physician or dietitian. Any application of the recommendations set forth in the following pages is at the reader's discretion. The reader should consult with his or her own physician or dietitian concerning the recommendations in this book.

Copyright © text 1997, 2000 Kaye Foster-Powell, Jennie Brand-Miller, Thomas M. S. Wolever, Stephen Colagiuri

First published in Australia in 1997 under the title *Pocket Guide to the G.I. Factor for People with Diabetes* by Hodder Headline Australia Pty Limited.

This edition is published by arrangement with Hodder Headline Australia Pty Limited.

Library of Congress Cataloging-in-Publication Data
Brand-Miller, Janette, 1952-
     The glucose revolution pocket guide to diabetes /
by Jennie Brand-Miller, Stephen Colagiuri, Kaye Foster-Powell.
     p. cm.
     First published in Australia in 1997 under the title: Pocket guide to the G.I. factor for people with diabetes by Kaye Foster-Powell, Jennie Brand-Miller, Stephen Colagiuri.
     ISBN 1-56924-675-0
     1. Glycemic index—Handbooks, manuals, etc.   2. Diabetes—Diet therapy—Handbooks, manuals, etc.   I. Title: Diabetes.   II. Colagiuri, Stephen.   III. Foster-Powell, Kaye.   IV. Foster-Powell, Kaye. Pocket guide to the G.I. factor for people with diabetes.   V. Title.

RC662.B715 2000
616.4'620654—dc21
                                                                  99-042191

9 8 7 6 5 4 3

Designed by Pauline Neuwirth, Neuwirth & Associates, Inc.
Distributed by Publishers Group West
Manufactured in the United States of America

CONTENTS

PREFACE

The Glucose Revolution is the definitive, all-in-one guide to the glycemic index. Now we have written this pocket guide to show you how the glycemic index (G.I.) can help you achieve better control of your diabetes. As we explain in *The Glucose Revolution*, the glycemic index:

- is a proven guide to the true physiological effects foods—especially carbohydrates—have on blood sugar levels;
- provides an easy and effective way to eat a healthy diet and control fluctuations in blood sugar.

This book offers more in-depth information about using the glycemic index to manage diabetes than we had room to include in *The Glucose Revolution*. Much new information appears in this book that is not in *The Glucose Revolution*, including the questions most frequently asked by diabetics about the glycemic index, a week's worth of low-G.I. meal plans, and success stories about diabetics who have made the switch to low G.I. foods—and in the processs have achieved better control of their blood glucose levels.

This book has been written to be read alongside *The Glucose Revolution*, so in the event you haven't already consulted that book, please be sure to do so, for a more comprehensive discussion of the glycemic index and all its uses.

Chapter 1

WHAT THIS BOOK CAN DO FOR YOU

THE IMPORTANCE OF A GOOD DIET

WHAT IS THE GLYCEMIC INDEX?

HOW TO USE THIS BOOK

D id you know that every day in the United States, more than 2,000 people are diagnosed with diabetes? And even more striking is the number of people who have the disease and *don't even know it*: In addition to the 10.3 million who have already been diagnosed with diabetes, another 5.4 million people remain undiagnosed—unaware that they're even sick!

In fact, many people don't even know they are suffering from the seventh leading cause of death in the United States until they develop one of its life-threatening complications such as blindness, kidney disease, heart disease, stroke or nerve damage.

■ ■ ■

THE IMPORTANCE OF A GOOD DIET

The good news? You can control many diabetic symptoms by getting regular medical check-ups, enjoying plenty of exercise and eating a healthy diet. That's how this book can help. Health authorities all over the world stress the importance of high carbohydrate diets for good health and diabetes management. The question now is which type of carbohydrate is best for people with diabetes? Research on the glycemic index (what we call the G.I.) shows that different carbohydrate foods have dramatically different effects on blood sugar levels.

■

THE GLYCEMIC INDEX GIVES YOU THE TRUE STORY ABOUT
THE CARBOHYDRATE—BLOOD SUGAR CONNECTION.
FOR PEOPLE WITH DIABETES THIS CAN MEAN A
NEW LEASE ON LIFE . . . LITERALLY!

■

Understanding the glycemic index has made an enormous difference to the diet and lifestyle of people with diabetes because the findings reveal that:

- many traditionally "taboo" foods don't cause the unfavorable effects on blood sugar they were believed to have;
- diets containing low G.I. foods improve blood sugar control in people with type 1 (insulin-dependent) and type 2 (non-insulin-dependent) diabetes;
- many more foods make up a healthy diet for someone with diabetes than was once believed.

WHAT IS THE GLYCEMIC INDEX?

The glycemic index is a ranking of foods based on their immediate effect on blood sugar levels. Carbohydrate foods that break down quickly during digestion have the highest G.I. values because their blood sugar response is fast and high. Carbohydrate foods that break down slowly, releasing glucose gradually into the bloodstream, have low G.I. values.

The rate of carbohydrate digestion has important implications for everybody. It's vital that people with diabetes learn about the glycemic index so they can base their diets on sound scientific evidence. (For more information about the glycemic index, see Chapter 5.)

HOW TO USE THIS BOOK

Many people with diabetes find that despite doing all they are told, their blood sugar levels remain too high. This book contains the most up-to-date information about carbohydrate and the optimum diet for people with diabetes. It explains which types of carbohydrate are best and why—information based on scientific research, clinical trials and the real experiences of real people. This Pocket Guide:

- shows you how to include more of the right type of carbohydrate in your diet;
- provides practical hints for meal preparation and tips to help you make the glycemic index work for you throughout the day;
- gives a week of low G.I. menus plus a nutritional analysis for each menu and its glycemic index;

- explains how scientists measure the glycemic index; and
- includes an A to Z listing of over 300 foods with their G.I., carbohydrate and fat counts.

Chapter 2

TREAT DIABETES WITH A LOW G.I. DIET

WHAT DOES THE GLYCEMIC INDEX MEAN
FOR PEOPLE WITH DIABETES?

WHY IS THE GLYCEMIC INDEX SO
IMPORTANT IN DIABETES?

THE KEY IS THE RATE OF DIGESTION

WHAT IS THE OPTIMUM DIET
FOR PEOPLE WITH DIABETES?

CHECKLIST: THE OPTIMUM DIET
FOR PEOPLE WITH DIABETES

One of the major aims of diabetes therapy is to maintain near normal blood sugar levels. Not long ago, people with diabetes were told to eat complex carbohydrates (starches) because it was believed they were slowly absorbed causing a smaller rise in blood sugar levels. Simple sugars were restricted because they were thought to be quickly absorbed and their blood sugar response would therefore be fast and high.

These assumptions were wrong! We now know that the concept of simple and complex carbohydrates doesn't tell us how carbohydrate will actually behave in the body. Different carbohydrate containing foods do have different effects on blood sugar levels, but we can't predict the effect by looking at the sugar or starch content.

WHAT DOES THE GLYCEMIC INDEX MEAN FOR PEOPLE WITH DIABETES?

Since the 1980s, scientists have studied the actual blood sugar responses to hundreds of different foods on healthy people and on people with diabetes. They gave them real foods and then measured the blood sugar levels at frequent intervals, for up to two to three hours after the meal. To compare foods according to their true physiological effect on blood sugar levels, they came up with the term "glycemic index" (G.I.). This is simply a ranking of foods from 0 to 100 that tells us whether a food will raise blood sugar levels dramatically, moderately, or just a little.

■

IT'S TIME TO FORGET ABOUT SIMPLE AND COMPLEX CARBOHYDRATE AND TO THINK IN TERMS OF LOW G.I. FOODS AND HIGH G.I. FOODS.

■

Research on the glycemic index has turned some widely held beliefs upside down. The first surprise was that many starchy foods (some types of bread and potato and many types of rice) are digested and absorbed very quickly—not slowly as we had always assumed. The second surprise was that moderate amounts of many sugary foods did not produce the dramatic rises in blood sugar that we had thought.

The truth was that many foods containing sugar actually showed intermediate blood sugar responses, often lower than some types of bread, for example.

So, you can forget the old distinctions that we used to make between starchy foods and sugary foods or simple versus complex carbohydrate. These distinctions have no scientific basis at all. The glycemic index tells the true story.

THE PANCREAS PRODUCES INSULIN

The pancreas is a vital organ near the stomach, and its main job is to produce the hormone insulin. Carbohydrate stimulates the secretion of insulin more than any other component of food. The slow absorption of the carbohydrate in our food means that the pancreas doesn't have to work so hard and needs to produce less insulin. If the pancreas is overstimulated over a long period of time, it may become "exhausted" and type 2 diabetes can develop in genetically susceptible people. Even without diabetes, high insulin levels are undesirable because they increase the risk of heart disease.

Unfortunately, over time, we have begun to eat more "refined" foods and fewer "whole" foods. This new way of eating has brought with it higher bood sugar levels after a meal and higher insulin responses, as well. Though our bodies do need insulin for carbohydrate metabolism, high levels of the hormone have a profound effect on the development of many diseases. In fact, medical experts now believe that high insulin levels are one of the key factors responsible for heart disease and hypertension. Insulin influences the way we metabolize foods, determining whether we burn fat or carbohydrate to meet our energy needs and ultimately determining whether we store fat in our bodies.

WHY IS THE GLYCEMIC INDEX SO IMPORTANT IN DIABETES MANAGEMENT?

If blood sugar levels are not properly controlled, diabetes can cause damage to the blood vessels in the heart, legs, brain, eyes and kidneys. For this reason, heart attacks, strokes, kidney failure and blindness are more common in people with diabetes. High blood sugar levels can also damage the nerves in the feet, which can cause pain, irritation and loss of sensation in the feet.

High insulin levels can also damage the blood vessels of the heart, legs and brain. In fact, some researchers think that high insulin levels might cause the muscle in the walls of blood vessels to thicken. This thickening would cause the blood vessels to narrow and slow the flow of blood. At that point, a clot could form and stop the blood flow altogether, causing a heart attack or stroke.

■

THE OPTIMUM DIET FOR PEOPLE WITH DIABETES CONTAINS A WIDE VARIETY OF FOODS.

■

In general, studies show an excellent correlation between the glycemic index of a food and its insulin response. With low G.I. foods, there's a reduced secretion of the hormone insulin over the course of the day. With high G.I. foods, the body produces larger amounts of insulin, resulting in higher levels of insulin in the blood.

It makes sense for people with type 2 or non-insulin-dependent diabetes to eat foods with low G.I. values to help control blood sugar levels, and do so with lower levels of insulin. (A low G.I. diet improves the body's sensitivity to insulin, so the insulin you do have works better.) This may have the added benefit of reducing the large vessel damage that accounts for many of the problems that diabetes can cause.

We also know that a low G.I. diet in conjunction with a low fat intake can help keep your blood vessels healthy by keeping your levels of blood fats down. Studies have shown that people have lower levels of blood fats (such as cholesterol and triglycerides) when they eat lower G.I. foods.

THE KEY IS THE RATE OF DIGESTION

Here's how digestion impacts the glycemic index of a food: Carbohydrate foods that break down quickly during digestion have the highest G.I. values. Conversely, carbohydrates that break down slowly, releasing glucose gradually into the bloodstream, have low G.I. values. (For most people most of the time, low G.I. foods have advantages over high G.I. foods.)

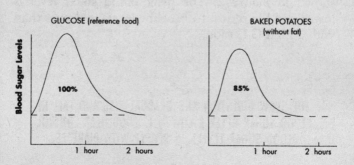

Figure 1. The effect of pure glucose (50 g) and baked potatoes without fat (50 g carbohydrate portion) on blood sugar levels.

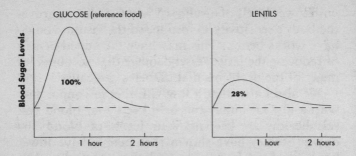

Figure 2. The effect of pure glucose (50 g) and lentils (50 g carbohydrate portion) on blood sugar levels.

The higher the glycemic index, the higher the blood sugar levels after consumption of the food. Rice Krispies (G.I. 82) and baked potatoes (G.I. 85) have very high G.I. values, meaning their effect on blood sugar levels is almost as high as that of an equal amount of pure glucose (yes, you read it correctly).

Figure 1 shows the blood sugar response to potatoes compared with pure glucose. Foods with a low glycemic index (such as lentils, with an average of 28) show a flatter blood sugar response when eaten, as shown in Figure 2. The peak blood sugar level is lower and the return to baseline levels is slower than with a high G.I. food.

■

THE SLOW DIGESTION AND GRADUAL RISE AND FALL IN BLOOD SUGAR AFTER A LOW G.I. FOOD HELP CONTROL BLOOD SUGAR LEVELS IN PEOPLE WITH DIABETES.

■

WHAT IS THE OPTIMUM DIET
FOR PEOPLE WITH DIABETES?

For over a hundred years, people with diabetes have been given advice on what to eat. Many diets were based more on unproven (although seemingly logical) theories, rather than actual research. In 1915, for example, the *Boston Medical and Surgical Journal* advocated that the best dietary treatment for someone with diabetes was "limitation of all components of the diet." This translated to a very low calorie diet interspersed with days of fasting. Unfortunately, malnutrition was often the result!

Fortunately, good quality scientific research supports today's dietary recommendations for people with diabetes. We now know that:

∎

A DIET THAT'S GOOD FOR PEOPLE WITH DIABETES IS A DIET THAT IS GOOD FOR EVERYONE.

∎

CHECKLIST: THE OPTIMUM DIET FOR PEOPLE WITH DIABETES

Eating a healthy diet is easy once you've mastered a few basic concepts. To manage your diabetes properly, you need to eat:

- **Plenty of whole grain cereals, breads, vegetables and fruits.** A low fat, low G.I. diet contains lots of dense heavy grain breads; cereals such as rice, barley, couscous, cracked wheat; legumes such as kidney beans and lentils; and all types of fruit and vegetables.

- **Only small amounts of fat, especially saturated fat.** Limit cookies, cakes, butter, potato chips, fried fast foods, whole milk dairy products and fatty meats and sausages, which are all high in saturated fat. Polyunsaturated and monounsaturated oils such as olive, canola and peanut are healthier types of fats.
- **A moderate amount of sugar and sugar containing foods.** It's okay to include your favorite sweetener or sweet food—small quantities of sugar, honey, syrup and jam—to make meals more palatable and enjoyable.
- **Only a moderate quantity of alcohol.** Limit your alcohol consumption to only 2 drinks (for men) and 1 drink (for women) per day, with at least 2 alcohol-free days a week.
- **Only a moderate amount of salt and salted foods.** Boost flavors by using lemon juice, fresh ground black pepper, garlic, chili, herbs and other seasonings rather than adding salt to your food.

■

CARBOHYDRATE IS THE ONLY PART OF FOOD THAT DIRECTLY AFFECTS BLOOD SUGAR LEVELS.

■

HOW DOES FOOD AFFECT OUR BLOOD SUGAR?

Our bodies burn fuel all the time, and the fuel our bodies like best is carbohydrate, which is the *only* fuel that the brain and red blood cells can use.

When we eat carbohydrate foods, the body breaks them down in the gut into a form that can be absorbed and used by the cells. This process is called digestion. Digestion starts in the mouth when amylase, the digestive enzyme in saliva, is incorporated into the food by chewing. The activity of this enzyme stops in the stomach. Most of the digestion continues only when the carbohydrate reaches the small intestine.

In the small intestine, amylase from pancreatic juice breaks down the large molecules of starch into short chain molecules. These and any disaccharide sugars are then broken into simpler monosaccharides by enzymes in the wall of the intestine. The monosaccharides that result—glucose, fructose and galactose—are absorbed from the small intestine into the bloodstream.

The body responds by releasing insulin, which clears the sugar from the blood by moving it into the muscles and cells where it is used for energy. Some glucose stays in the blood to serve the brain and central nervous system.

There are still people who think that because carbohydrate raises blood sugar, people who have diabetes should not eat it at all. This is wrong: Carbohydrate is a necessary part of a healthy diet. For people with diabetes, choosing carbohydrate foods with a low glycemic index flattens out the peaks and valleys in blood sugar and helps achieve more stable blood sugar levels.

- People with type 1 or insulin-dependent diabetes need to balance the amount and timing of carbohydrate in their diet with their dose of insulin and their activity level (rarely an easy task).
- People with type 2 or non-insulin-dependent diabetes, who have a relative lack of insulin, should distribute their carbohydrate intake throughout the day and may need to consider the timing of their meals in relation to any diabetes medications they take.

AT LEAST HALF OF OUR TOTAL DAILY CALORIES SHOULD COME FROM CARBOHYDRATE.

Chapter 3

8 DIABETES MYTHS— DISPELLED

SUGAR ISN'T NECESSARILY BAD

ALL CARBOHYDRATES ARE NOT CREATED EQUAL

STARCHY FOODS AREN'T FATTENING

AND MORE . . .

*R*esearch into the glycemic index shows that some of the popular beliefs about food and diabetes just aren't true. Below, we separate the facts from the fallacies.

MYTH 1: SUGAR IS THE WORST THING FOR PEOPLE WITH DIABETES.

There is absolute consensus that sugar does not cause diabetes. Sugar and sugary foods in normal portions have no greater effect on blood sugar levels than many starchy foods. Saturated fat is far worse for people with diabetes.

■ Type 1 diabetes (insulin-dependent diabetes) is

an autoimmune health problem triggered by unknown environmental factors—possibly viruses.

- Type 2 diabetes (non-insulin-dependent diabetes) is strongly inherited but lifestyle factors such as lack of exercise and overweight increase the risk of developing it. Because the dietary treatment of diabetes in the past involved strict avoidance of sugar, many people wrongly believed that sugar was in some way implicated as a cause of the disease.

MYTH 2: ALL COMPLEX CARBOHYDRATES OR STARCHES ARE SLOWLY DIGESTED IN THE INTESTINE.

Not true. Some starch, such as that in mashed potatoes, is digested quickly, causing a greater change in blood sugar level than many sugar-containing foods.

MYTH 3: STARCHY FOODS SUCH AS BREAD AND POTATOES ARE FATTENING.

Not true. Bread and potatoes are carbohydrate (fuel) foods—the types of foods your body burns most readily. They are the least likely to be stored as body fat.

MYTH 4: EATING A LOT OF SUGAR CAUSES DIABETES.

Not true. A diet high in fat and quickly digested carbohydrates contributes to obesity, which makes type 2 diabetes more likely to appear in those who are at risk.

MYTH 5: YOU CAN'T LOSE WEIGHT EATING BETWEEN MEAL SNACKS.

Not true. The type and total amount of calories consumed and the amount of calories the body uses determine body weight. You can safely include low fat, high carbohydrate snacks in a low calorie eating plan.

MYTH 6: SUGAR IS FATTENING.

Not true. Sugar is just another carbohydrate, and it's almost impossible to turn it into body fat.

MYTH 7: HIGH BLOOD SUGAR IS CAUSED BY EATING TOO MUCH SUGAR.

Not true. A number of factors can cause blood sugar levels to rise including the body's response to stress or illness, reduced activity, missed medications and excess carbohydrate.

MYTH 8: SUGAR IN THE DIET WILL RESULT IN LOWER INTAKES OF VITAMINS AND MINERALS.

Not true. Studies show that diets containing moderate amounts of refined sugars are perfectly healthy (10 to 12 percent of calories) and the sugar helps make many nutritious foods (oatmeal, for example) more palatable. Diets high in natural sugar from a range of sources, including dairy foods and fruit, often have higher levels of micronutrients such as calcium, riboflavin and vitamin C.

Chapter 4

ASSESS YOUR CARBOHYDRATE NEEDS

5 KEYS TO A HEALTHY DIET

HOW MUCH CARBOHYDRATE DO YOU NEED?

*Y*our calorie (and carbohydrate) requirements depend on your age, gender, activity level and body size; it's not possible to publish standard figures that will apply to everyone. If you want to assess your own specific calorie requirements and calculate exactly how much carbohydrate you need, we suggest that you consult a dietitian. To find a registered dietitian near you, turn to page 125.

Once you have the amount of carbohydrate in your diet right, the next step is to choose the *right type* of carbohydrate foods—those with low G.I. values.

■ ■ ■

5 KEYS TO A HEALTHY DIET

- Eat carbohydrate-rich foods at every meal and make sure that carbohydrates and vegetables form a large proportion of the meal. (Together, they should cover 75 percent of your plate.)
- Eat carbohydrate-rich foods for snacks, rather than high fat foods.
- Include at least the minimum quantity of carbohydrate foods suggested for small eaters (see "Carbohydrate Requirements" on page 20).
- Make at least half your carbohydrate choices be foods with low G.I. values.
- Don't eat too much protein or fat. High fat foods are a concentrated source of calories, and it takes only a little extra of them to throw your diet out of balance.

THE SUGAR-FAT SEESAW

Did you know that fat and sugar tend to show a reciprocal or seesaw relationship in the diet? Research shows that diets high in fat are low in sugar, and diets low in fat are high in sugar. But studies over the past decade have found that diets high in sugar are no less nutritious than low sugar diets. This is because restricting sugar is frequently followed by higher fat consumption, and most fatty foods are poor sources of nutrients.

In some cases, high sugar diets have been found to have higher micronutrient contents. This is because sugar is often used to sweeten some very nutritious foods, such as yogurts, breakfast cereals and milk.

A low sugar (and high fat) diet has more proven disadvantages than a high sugar (and low fat) diet.

■

TO IMPROVE THE QUALITY OF OUR DIET MOST OF US
NEED TO EAT MORE CARBOHYDRATE AND LESS FAT.

■

HOW MUCH CARBOHYDRATE DO YOU NEED?

About half of our total calorie intake should come
from carbohydrate. We need to consume 125 grams
(g) of carbohydrate for every 1000 calories.

- For a low calorie diet (1200 calories), it means
  eating about 150 g of carbohydrate per day
  (equivalent to 10 slices of bread).
- For a young, active person with higher energy
  requirements (around 2000 calories), it means
  eating 250 g of carbohydrate per day (equivalent to 17 slices of bread).

We have calculated sample carbohydrate intakes
for both small and bigger eaters.

■

A HEALTHY DIET IS HIGH IN CARBOHYDRATE
AND LOW IN FAT.

■

CARBOHYDRATE REQUIREMENTS
FOR SMALL EATERS

You might consider yourself a small eater if you:

- are a small-framed female
- have a small appetite
- do very little physical activity
- are trying to lose weight

Even the smallest eater needs these carbohydrate foods every day. This food list supplies 188 g of carbohydrate, suitable for a 1,500 calorie diet.

- about 4 slices of bread (4 ozs.) or the equivalent (crackers, rolls, English muffins)

PLUS

- about 3 small pieces of fruit or the equivalent (fresh, canned, dried)

PLUS

- 1 cup of high carbohydrate (starchy) vegetables (corn, legumes, potato, sweet potato)

PLUS

- at least 1 cup of breakfast cereal or grain (cooked rice or pasta, barley, quinoa or other grain)

PLUS

- 2 cups of low fat milk or the equivalent (yogurt, ice cream). This includes milk in your tea and coffee and with your cereal

---

CARBOHYDRATE REQUIREMENTS
FOR BIGGER EATERS

You're a bigger eater if you are:

- an active young female of average frame size
- doing regular physical activity (but not prolonged strenuous exercise)
- an active adult male or teenage boy
- working as a laborer

The following food list provides 313 g of carbohydrate which is suitable for a 2,500 calorie diet.

- about 6 slices of bread (6 ozs.) or the equivalent (crackers, rolls, English muffins)

PLUS

- about 3 medium sized pieces of fruit or the equivalent (fresh, canned, dried)

PLUS

- 2 cups of high carbohydrate vegetables (corn, legumes, potato, sweet potato) and at least 1 cup of raw vegetables

PLUS

- at least 2 cups of cereal or grain food (breakfast cereal or cooked rice, or pasta or other grain)

PLUS

- 2 cups of low fat milk or the equivalent (yogurt, ice cream). This includes milk in your tea and coffee and with your cereal

Chapter 5

SOME BACKGROUND ON THE GLYCEMIC INDEX

WHAT IS THE GLYCEMIC INDEX?

THE GLYCEMIC INDEX MADE SIMPLE

MEASURING THE GLYCEMIC INDEX

WHAT IS THE GLYCEMIC INDEX?

The glycemic index of foods is simply a ranking of foods based on their immediate effect on blood sugar levels. To make a fair comparison, all foods are compared with a reference food such as pure glucose and are tested in equivalent carbohydrate amounts. The glycemic index is a scientifically validated tool in the dietary management of diabetes and weight reduction.

Originally, research into the glycemic index of foods was inspired by the desire to identify the best foods for people with diabetes. But scientists are now discovering that the glycemic index has implications for everyone.

Today we know the glycemic index of hundreds of different food items—both generic and name-brand—that have been tested following a standardized testing method. The tables in Chapter 20 (pages 111 to 123) give the glycemic index of a range of common foods, including many tested at the University of Toronto and the University of Sydney.

THE GLYCEMIC INDEX MADE SIMPLE

As we mentioned in Chapter 2, carbohydrate foods that break down quickly during digestion have the highest G.I. values. The blood glucose, or sugar, response is fast and high. In other words the glucose in the bloodstream increases rapidly. On the other hand, carbohydrates that break down slowly, releasing glucose gradually into the bloodstream, have low G.I. values. An analogy might be the popular fable of the tortoise and the hare. The hare, just like high G.I. foods, speeds away full steam ahead but loses the race to the tortoise with his slow and steady pace. Similarly, slow and steady low G.I. foods produce a smooth blood sugar curve without wild fluctuations.

For most people most of the time, the foods with a low glycemic index have advantages over those with high G.I. values. Figure 3 shows the effect of slow and fast carbohydrate on blood sugar levels.

The substance that produces the greatest rise in blood sugar levels is pure glucose itself. All other foods have less effect when fed in equal amounts of carbohydrate. The glycemic index of pure glucose is set at 100, and every other food is ranked on a scale from 0 to 100 according to its actual effect on blood sugar levels.

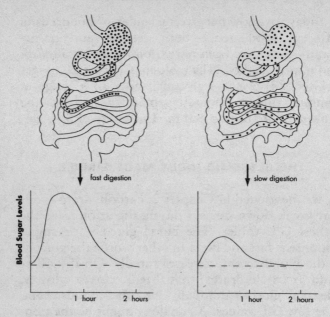

Figure 3. Slow and fast carbohydrate digestion and the consequent levels of sugar in the blood.

The glycemic index of a food cannot be predicted from its composition or the glycemic index of related foods. To test the glycemic index, you need real people and real foods. We describe how the glycemic index of a food is measured in the following section. There is no easy, inexpensive substitute test. Scientists always follow standardized methods so that results from one group of people can be directly compared with those of another group.

In total, eight to ten people need to be tested and the glycemic index of the food is the average value of the group. We know this average figure is reproducible and that a different group of volunteers will produce a similar result. Results obtained in a group of people with diabetes are comparable to those without diabetes.

The most important point to note is that all foods are tested in equivalent carbohydrate amounts. For example, 100 grams of bread (about 3½ slices of sandwich bread) is tested because this contains 50 grams of carbohydrate. Likewise, 60 grams of jelly beans (containing 50 grams of carbohydrate) is compared with the reference food. We know how much carbohydrate is in a food by consulting food composition tables, the manufacturer's data or measuring it ourselves in the laboratory.

■

THE GLYCEMIC INDEX IS A CLINICALLY PROVEN TOOL IN ITS APPLICATIONS TO DIABETES, APPETITE CONTROL AND REDUCING THE RISK OF HEART DISEASE.

■

MEASURING THE GLYCEMIC INDEX

Scientists use just six steps to determine the glycemic index of a food. Simple as this may sound, it's actually quite a time-consuming process. Here's how it works.

1. An amount of food containing 50 grams of carbohydrate is given to a volunteer to eat. For example, to test boiled spaghetti, the volunteer would be given 200 grams of spaghetti, which supplies 50 grams of carbohydrate (we work this out from food composition tables)—50 grams of carbohydrate is equivalent to 3 tablespoons of pure glucose powder.

2. Over the next two hours (or three hours if the

volunteer has diabetes), we take a sample of their blood every 15 minutes during the first hour and every 30 minutes thereafter. The blood sugar level of these blood samples is measured in the laboratory and recorded.

3. The blood sugar level is plotted on a graph and the area under the curve is calculated using a computer program (Figure 4).

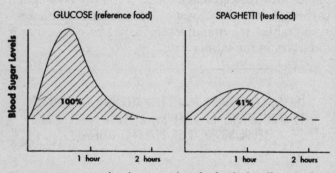

Figure 4. Measuring the glycemic index of a food. The effect of a food on blood sugar levels is calculated using the area under the curve (shaded area). The area under the curve after consumption of the test food is compared with the same area after the reference food (usually 50 grams of pure glucose or a 50 gram carbohydrate portion of white bread).

4. The volunteer's response to spaghetti (or whatever food is being tested) is compared with his or her blood sugar response to 50 grams of pure glucose (the reference food).

5. The reference food is tested on two or three separate occasions and an average value is calculated. This is done to reduce the effect of day-to-day variation in blood sugar responses.

6. The average glycemic index found in eight to ten people is the glycemic index of that food.

5 KEY FACTORS THAT INFLUENCE
THE GLYCEMIC INDEX

Cooking methods

Cooking and processing increases the glycemic index of a food because it increases the amount of gelatinized starch in the food. Cornflakes are one example.

Physical form of the food

An intact fibrous coat, such as that on grains and legumes, acts as a physical barrier and slows down digestion, lowering a food's G.I. value.

Type of starch

There are two types of starch in foods, amylose and amylopectin. The more amylose starch a food contains, the lower the glycemic index.

Fiber

Viscous, soluble fibers, such as those found in rolled oats and apples, slow down digestion and lower a food's glycemic index.

Sugar

The presence of sugar, as well as the type of sugar, will influence a food's glycemic index. Fruits with a low glycemic index, such as apples and oranges, are high in fructose.

Chapter 6

OUR DIETS NEED AN OVERHAUL

TOO MUCH FAT

WHY WE NEED TO EAT MORE
CARBOHYDRATE

WHAT IS A BALANCED DIET?

Today's Western diet is the product of industrialization based on inventions ranging from Jethro Tull's seed drill (in 1701) to the high speed steel roller mills for milling cereals (in the nineteenth century) and advances in processing food to give it a longer shelf life. The benefits are many: We have plenty of relatively cheap, palatable and safe foods available, and gone are the days of monotonous fare, gaps in the food supply and weevil-infested and adulterated food. Also long gone are widespread vitamin deficiencies such as scurvy and pellagra. Today's food manufacturers work hard to bring us irresistible products that meet the demands of both gourmets and health conscious consumers.

Many of the new foods are still based on our staple cereals—wheat, corn, and oats—but the original grain has been ground down to produce fine flours that yield the best quality breads, cakes, cookies, breakfast cereals and snack foods.

Cereal chemists and bakers know that the finest particle size flour produces the most palatable and shelf-stable end products. But this striving for excellence in one area has resulted in unforeseen problems in another. Today's staple carbohydrate foods, including some ordinary breads, are quickly digested and absorbed, and the resulting effect on blood sugar levels has created a problem for many of us.

∎

TRADITIONAL DIETS ALL AROUND THE WORLD CONTAINED SLOWLY DIGESTED AND ABSORBED CARBOHYDRATE——LOW G.I. FOODS. IN CONTRAST, MODERN DIETS WITH THEIR QUICKLY DIGESTED FINE WHITE FLOURS ARE BASED ON HIGH G.I. FOODS.

∎

TOO MUCH FAT

The other undesirable aspect of the modern diet is its high fat content. Food manufacturers, bakers and chefs know we love to eat fat. We love its creaminess and mouth feel and find it easy to consume in excess. It makes our meat more tender, our vegetables and salads more palatable and our sweet foods even tastier. We prefer potatoes as French fries or potato chips, to have our fish battered and fried, and our pastas in rich creamy sauces. With a wave of the fat wand,

bland high carbohydrate foods such as rice and oats
are magically transformed into delicious, calorie-
laden foods such as fried rice and sweetened granola.
In fact, when you analyze it, much of our diet today
is an unwanted but delicious combination of both fat
and quickly digested carbohydrate.

WHAT'S WRONG WITH OUR
WAY OF EATING?

- The modern diet is too high in saturated fat and quick-
  release carbohydrate.
- The carbohydrate we eat is digested and absorbed too
  quickly because most modern starchy foods have a high
  glycemic index.

WHY WE NEED TO EAT MORE CARBOHYDRATE

For once, health experts are nearly unanimous. Most
agree that the food we eat for breakfast, lunch and
dinner and for those in-between snacks should be
low in fat and high in carbohydrate. The same diet
that helps prevent our becoming overweight also
reduces our risk of developing heart disease, diabetes
and many types of cancer. (This same high carbohydrate and low fat diet also improves athletic performance. For more information on that subject, read
our companion guide, *The Glucose Revolution
Pocket Guide to Sports Nutrition*.)

But the story doesn't end there. To reduce the fat
content of our diet, we need to eat more carbohydrate. In fact, carbohydrate should be the main
source of calories in our food—not fat. Carbohydrate

and fat have a reciprocal relationship in our diets: If we eat more high carbohydrate foods, they tend to displace the high fat foods from our diet. The new emphasis on eating lots of high carbohydrate foods has focused attention on the differences among carbohydrates.

WHAT IS A BALANCED DIET?

It makes sense to balance our food intake with the rate our bodies use it in order to maintain a steady weight. These days, however, this balance is difficult to achieve, since it's so easy to overeat. Refined foods, convenience foods and fast foods frequently lack fiber and conceal fat so that before we feel full, we have overdosed on calories. It is even easier not to exercise. It takes longer to walk somewhere than it does to drive (except perhaps in rush hour). With intake exceeding output on a regular basis, the result for too many of us is gaining weight.

We need to adapt our lifestyle to our high caloric diet and fewer physical demands. It's become very important to catch bursts of physical activity wherever we can to increase our energy output. (See the following chapter for more information on exercise.)

While you work on increasing your energy output, the glycemic index can help you select the best foods to balance your intake. Its high carbohydrate basis ensures a filling diet that isn't packed with calories.

Chapter 7

THE BENEFITS OF LIVING AN ACTIVE LIFE

THE BENEFITS OF EXERCISE

HOW TO GET MOVING

USING THE GLYCEMIC INDEX
WHEN YOU EXERCISE

8 WAYS TO MAKE EXERCISE WORK FOR YOU

*D*iet isn't the only way to manage diabetes. Because the disease stays with you for the rest of your life, taking good care of yourself requires adopting a few healthy lifestyle habits that must last a lifetime.

A multitude of changes in our living habits now mean that in both work and recreation we are more sedentary than ever. Our physical activity levels are now so low that we take in more calories than we burn off, causing us to gain weight. Luckily, exercise is our ticket back to healthy living.

Regular physical activity can reduce our blood sugar levels, lower our risk of heart and blood vessel disease, lower high blood pressure, increase stamina, reduce stress and help us relax. It's a good idea for all of us.

■

To lose weight you need to eat fewer calories and burn more calories—and that means getting regular exercise and leading a more active lifestyle.

■

THE BENEFITS OF EXERCISE

Most people could tell you at least one health benefit of exercise (reduces blood pressure, lowers the risk of heart disease, improves circulation, increases stamina, flexibility and strength), but the most motivating aspect of exercise is feeling so good about yourself for doing it.

Exercise speeds up our metabolic rate. By increasing our caloric expenditure, exercise helps to balance our sometimes excessive caloric intake from food.

More movement makes our muscles better at using fat as a source of fuel. By improving the way insulin works, exercise increases the amount of fat we burn.

A low G.I. diet has the same effect. Low G.I. foods reduce the amount of insulin we need, which makes fat easier to burn and harder to store. Since it's body fat that you want to get rid of when you lose weight, exercise in combination with a low G.I. diet makes a lot of sense!

HOW TO GET MOVING

Getting more exercise doesn't necessarily mean daily aerobics classes and jogging around the block (although this is great if you want to do it). What it *does* mean is moving more in everyday living. It's the day-to-day things we do—shopping, ironing, chasing kids, walking from the train station—where we spend the bulk of our energy.

Since so much of our lifestyle is designed now to reduce our physical exertion, it's become very important to catch bursts of physical activity wherever we can, to increase our energy output. It may mean using the stairs instead of the elevator, taking a 10 minute walk at lunch time, trotting on a treadmill while you watch the news or talk on the telephone, walking to the grocery store to get the Sunday paper, hiding the remote control, parking a half mile from work or taking the dog for a walk each night. Whatever it means, do it. Even housework burns calories!

HOW EXERCISE KEEPS YOU MOVING

The effect of exercise doesn't stop when you do. People who exercise have higher metabolic rates, so their bodies continue to burn more calories every minute, even when they're asleep!

Besides increasing the incidental activity, you will also benefit from some planned aerobic activity, which causes you to breathe more heavily and makes your heart beat faster. Walking, cycling, swimming and stair climbing are just a few examples. You'll need to accumulate a total of at least 30 minutes of this type of activity 5 to 6 days a week.

Remember that reduction in body weight takes time. Even after you've made changes in your exercise habits, your weight may not be any different on the scale. (This is particularly true for women, whose bodies tend to adapt to increased caloric expenditure.)

Whatever it takes for you to burn more calories, do it. Try to regard movement as an opportunity to improve your physical well-being—not as an inconvenience.

USING THE GLYCEMIC INDEX WHEN YOU EXERCISE

We're talking about the everyday sort of moderate exercise that all of us should be doing. If you train physically hard a number of days a week and perhaps compete in sports you should read *The Glucose Revolution Pocket Guide to Sports Nutrition.*

It is sometimes necessary with diabetes to eat extra carbohydrate when you exercise depending on the type of diabetes you have and the type and amount of medication you take. Often, you won't want to increase your food intake—because the exercise is intended to burn off some earlier overconsumption! (For people with insulin-dependent diabetes, remember this will only work if you have enough insulin in your body and your blood sugars aren't too high to start with.)

You may need extra carbohydrate before you exercise, or, if the exercise is prolonged over an hour or more, you may need extra carbohydrate while you exercise, too. Whether or not you need to eat extra and how much to take depends on your blood sugar level before, during and after the exercise and how your body responds to the exercise—all of which you learn from experience. Discuss your situation and how best to manage it with a dietitian, diabetes educator or doctor.

If you need to eat immediately before exercise to bring your blood sugar up, it makes sense to eat some high G.I. carbohydrate, such as a slice of regular bread, a couple of cookies or a ripe banana.

If you plan to eat your last meal or snack one to two hours before your exercise, it makes sense to eat a low G.I. meal to sustain you through the exercise, such as a sandwich made with low G.I. bread, a container of yogurt or an apple.

If you need to eat something quickly after or during exercise to restore your blood sugar level, use high G.I. food—crispbread or rice cakes, a bowl of cornflakes or Rice Krispies or a slice of watermelon, for example.

NOTE: Always remember to measure your blood sugar when you exercise to assess your body's response and judge your carbohydrate needs.

■

EXERCISE MAKES OUR MUSCLES BETTER AT USING FAT AS A SOURCE OF FUEL.

■

8 WAYS TO MAKE EXERCISE WORK FOR YOU

Your exercise routine will bring you lots of benefits if
you can:
1. see how it benefits you
2. enjoy what you do
3. feel that you can do it fairly well
4. fit it in with your daily life
5. keep it inexpensive
6. make it accessible
7. stay safe while doing it
8. make it socially acceptable to your peers

Chapter 8

YOUR NUTRIENT COUNTER

BREADS/CEREALS/GRAINS

VEGETABLES

FRUIT

DAIRY FOODS

MEAT AND ALTERNATIVES

To meet your average daily nutrient requirements you need to eat a certain amount of different types of foods. If you are trying to reduce your caloric intake there is still a minimum amount of certain foods that you should be eating each day. These are:

BREADS/CEREALS/AND GRAIN FOODS— 6 SERVINGS OR MORE

1 serving means:
- 1 bowl breakfast cereal (1 ounce)
- ½ cup cooked pasta or rice

- ½ cup cooked grain such as barley or wheat
- 1 slice bread
- ½ roll or muffin

VEGETABLES—3 SERVINGS

1 serving means:
- 1 medium potato (about 5 ounces)
- ½ cup cooked vegetables such as broccoli or carrot (2 ounces)
- 1 cup raw leafy vegetables, such as lettuce

FRUIT—2-4 SERVINGS

1 serving means:
- 1 medium orange (7 ounces)
- 1 medium apple (5 ounces)
- ½ cup strawberries (4 ounces)

DAIRY FOODS—2 SERVINGS

1 serving means:
- 8 ounces low fat milk
- 1½ ounces low fat cheese
- 8 ounces low fat yogurt

MEAT AND ALTERNATIVES—2 SERVINGS

1 serving means:
- 3 ounces cooked lean beef, veal, lamb or pork
- 3 ounces lean chicken (cooked, excluding bone)

- 3 ounces fish (cooked, excluding bone)
- 2 eggs
- ½ cup cooked beans

If you prefer larger servings of meat, go ahead, just make sure it's lean. Protein is a very satiating nutrient.

Chapter 9

HOW WELL ARE YOU EATING NOW?

DO YOU EAT ENOUGH CARBOHYDRATE?

IS YOUR DIET TOO HIGH IN FAT?

HOW DID YOU RATE?

*Y*ou can check the nutritional quality of your diet yourself; all you need is a record of your usual food intake. It is ideal if you can keep a food diary of everything you eat and drink for three to five days and use this for your assessment. Remember you have to eat as freely as you normally do, and write down everything—otherwise you're only cheating yourself!

Once you have your total food intake record complete, use the following serving size guidelines to check whether you have a balanced intake. The checklists on the following pages can be used to assess your carbohydrate and fat intake.

DO YOU EAT ENOUGH CARBOHYDRATE?

Looking at your diet record and using the serving size guide below estimate the number of servings of carbohydrate foods you had each day. For example, if you had a banana, 2 slices of bread and a medium potato, this counts as 4 servings of carbohydrate.

CARBOHYDRATE FOOD	ONE SERVING IS	HOW MANY DID YOU EAT?
Fruit	a handful or 1 medium piece	
Juice	about ¾ cup (6 ozs.)	
Dried fruit	¼ cup	
Bread	1 slice	
English muffin, roll, bagel	½ roll, muffin or small bagel	
Crackers, crispbread	2 large pieces or 3-4 plain crackers	
Rice cakes	2 rice cakes	
Muffin, cookies	½ muffin or 2 cookies	
Health bar/sports bar	approximately ½ average bar	
Breakfast cereal	1 bowl (1 oz.)	
Oatmeal	about ½ cup cooked cereal	
Rice	½ cup cooked rice	
Pasta, noodles	½ cup cooked noodles	
Pancakes	1 pancake, 4 inch	
Bulgur, couscous	about ⅓ cup, cooked	
Potato, sweet potato	1 small potato, about 3 ozs.	
Sweet corn	1 small ear or ½ cup kernels	
Lentils	⅓ cup, cooked	
Baked beans, other beans	about ½ cup, cooked	
Total		

Average the number of servings over all the days to come up with a daily average.

LOW G.I. EATING

Low G.I. eating means making a move back to the high carbohydrate foods that are staples in many parts of the world, especially whole grains (barley, oats, dried peas and beans) in combination with breads, pasta, vegetables, fruits and certain types of rice.

HOW DID YOU RATE?

- **Less than 4 servings a day:** Poor.
- **Between 4 and 8 servings a day:** Fair, but you need to eat a lot more.
- **Between 9 and 12 servings a day:** Good, could need more if you are hungry.
- **Between 13 and 16 servings a day:** Great—this should meet the needs of most people.

IS YOUR DIET TOO HIGH IN FAT?

Use this fat counter to tally up how much fat your diet contains. Do a tally for each day and then take an average. Using this fat counter you will need to compare the serving size listed with your serving size and multiply the grams of fat up or down to match your serving size. For example, if you estimate you might consume 2 cups of regular milk in a day, this supplies you with 16 grams of fat.

■ ■ ■

FOOD	FAT CONTENT (GRAMS)	HOW MUCH DID YOU EAT?
Dairy Foods		
Milk (8 ozs.) 1 cup		
whole	8	
2%	5	
nonfat	0	
Yogurt (8 ozs.)		
whole milk	7	
nonfat	0	
Ice cream, 2 scoops (1 cup)		
regular	15	
low fat	3	
fat free	0	
Cheese		
American, block cheese, 1 oz. slice	9	
reduced fat American cheese, 1 oz. slice	7	
low fat slices (per slice)	3	
cottage, small curd, 2 tablespoons	3	
ricotta, whole milk, 2 tablespoons	2	
Cream, 1 tablespoon		
heavy	6	
light	5	
Sour cream, 1 tablespoon		
regular	3	
light	1	
Fats and Oils		
Butter, 1 teaspoon	4	
Oil, any type, 1 tablespoon (½ oz.)	14	
Cooking spray, per spray	0	
Mayonnaise, 1 tablespoon	11	
Salad dressing, 1 tablespoon	6	

FOOD	FAT CONTENT (GRAMS)	HOW MUCH DID YOU EAT?
Meat		
Beef		
steak, flank, lean only, 3½ ozs.	10	
ground beef, extra-lean, 1 cup, 3½ ozs., cooked, drained	16	
sausage, frankfurter, grilled, 2 ozs.	16	
top sirloin, lean only, 3½ ozs.	8	
Lamb		
rib chop, grilled, lean only, 3½ ozs.	10	
leg, roasted, lean only, 3½ ozs.	7	
loin chop, grilled, lean only, 3 ½ ozs.	8	
Pork		
bacon, 3 strips, panfried	9	
ham, 1 slice, leg, lean, 3½ ozs.	5	
steak, lean only, 3½ ozs.	4	
leg, roasted, lean only, 3½ ozs.	9	
loin chop, lean only, 3½ ozs.	4	
Chicken		
breast, skinless, 3 ozs.	4	
drumstick, skinless, 2 ozs.	3	
thigh, skinless, 2 ozs.	6	
½ barbecue chicken (including skin)	30	
Fish		
grilled fish, 1 average fillet, 4 ozs.	1	
salmon, 3 ozs.	3	
fish sticks, frozen, 4 baked	14	
fish fillets, 2, batter-dipped, frozen, oven-baked, 6 ozs.		
regular	26	
light	10	
Snack Foods		
Chocolate bar, Hershey, 1½ ozs.	13	
Potato chips, 1 oz. bag	10	

FOOD	FAT CONTENT (GRAMS)	HOW MUCH DID YOU EAT?
Corn chips, 1 oz. bag	10	
Peanuts, ½ cup, (2½ ozs.)	35	
French fries, 25 pieces	20	
Pizza, cheese, 2 slices, medium pizza	22	
Pie, apple, snack size	15	
Popcorn, fat and salt added, 3 cups	9	
Total		

HOW DID YOU RATE?

- **Less than 40 grams:** Excellent. 30 to 40 grams of fat per day is recommended for those people trying to lose weight.
- **41 to 60 grams:** Good. A fat intake in this range is recommended for most adult men and women.
- **61 to 80 grams:** Acceptable if you are very active (doing hard physical work or athletic training). It is probably too much if you are trying to lose weight.
- **More than 80 grams:** You're probably eating too much fat, unless you're Superman or Superwoman!

Chapter 10

SECRETS TO LOW G.I. SNACKING

17 SUSTAINING SNACKS
5 SNACKING TIPS

*M*any people with diabetes need between-meal snacks to keep their blood sugar levels from dipping too low. The glycemic index is especially important when you eat carbohydrate by itself and not as part of a mixed meal, because carbohydrate tends to have a stronger effect on our blood sugar level when it is eaten alone.

When choosing a between-meal bite, pick a low-fat snack with a low glycemic index. For example, an apple with a glycemic index of 38 is better than a slice of white bread with a glycemic index of around 70, because it will cause a smaller jump in blood sugar levels.

New evidence suggests that the people who graze, eating small amounts of food throughout the day at frequent intervals, may actually be doing themselves a favor. Spreading the food out over longer periods of time will flatten out the peaks and valleys of blood glucose levels. So, snacking may be a good idea if you have diabetes—as long as you don't overeat and gain weight.

Some snack foods with a very low glycemic index (such as peanuts, at 14) have a very high fat content and are not recommended for people with a weight problem. As an occasional snack they are fine, especially because their fat is the healthier monounsaturated type. Just don't indulge in them every day. Remember, with peanuts, it's often hard to stop at just a handful!

17 SUSTAINING SNACKS

- An apple
- An apple and oat bran muffin
- Dried apricots
- A mini can of baked beans
- A small bowl of cherries
- Ice cream (low fat) in a cone
- Milk, milkshake or smoothie (low fat, of course)
- Oatmeal cookies, 2 to 3
- An orange
- 6 ounces of orange juice, freshly squeezed
- Pita bread spread with apple butter
- A big bowl of low fat popcorn
- One or 2 slices of raisin toast
- Whole grain bread sandwich with your favorite filling
- A bowl of Raisin Bran™ with skim milk
- A small box of raisins
- 6 to 8 ounces of light yogurt

5 SNACKING TIPS

- It is important to include a couple servings of dairy foods each day for your calcium needs. If you haven't used yogurt or cheese in any meals, you may choose to make a low fat milkshake. One or 2 scoops of low fat ice cream or pudding can also boost your daily calcium intake.
- If you like whole grain breads, an extra slice makes a very good choice for a snack. Other snacks can include toasted sourdough English muffin halves, a waffle or a slice of raisin bread with a little butter.
- Fruit is always a low calorie option for snacks. You should try to consume at least 3 servings a day. It may be helpful to prepare fruit in advance to make it accessible and easy to eat.
- Ryvita™ whole grain crispbreads are a low calorie snack if you want something dry and crunchy. Popcorn (prepared at home using a minimum of fat) is another good alternative.
- Keep vegetables (such as celery and carrot sticks, baby tomatoes, florets of blanched cauliflower or broccoli) ready prepared.

Chapter 11

STOCKING YOUR LOW G.I. PANTRY

BREADS

BREAKFAST CEREALS

RICE AND GRAINS

LEGUMES

VEGETABLES

FRUITS

DAIRY FOODS

USEFUL FLAVORINGS, SAUCES
AND DRESSINGS

HYPOGLYCEMIA: THE EXCEPTION TO
THE LOW G.I. RULE

*M*ake your low G.I. choices easier by keeping the right foods in your cupboard and refrigerator. Here's a starter list for you to follow.

BREADS

If you're the only one in the house who will eat the "birdseed bread," keep a loaf in the freezer and pull out slices as you need them. All of the breads below are made from whole grain flours.

■ ■ ■

- 100% stoneground whole wheat
- Arnold's rye
- Banana bread
- Chapati (Baisen)
- Natural Ovens 100% Whole Grain
- Natural Ovens Happiness
- Natural Ovens Hunger Filler
- Natural Ovens Natural Wheat
- Sourdough
- Sourdough rye
- Whole grain pumpernickel
- Whole wheat pita

**Natural Ovens breads are available in the United States through mail order. See "For More Information" on page 127 for ordering information.

BREAKFAST CEREALS

- Kellogg's All-Bran with extra fiber™
- Kellogg's Bran Buds with Psyllium™
- Muesli (low fat varieties, read the labels)
- Rolled or old-fashioned oats
- Oat bran
- Rice bran
- Oatmeal

RICE AND GRAINS

- Pearled barley
- Basmati rice, brown or long-grain rice
- Uncle Ben's Converted™ Rice
- Pasta of various shapes and flavors

LEGUMES

- Cooked lentils (red or brown), chickpeas, split peas
- Dried lentils, chickpeas, cannellini beans
- A variety of canned legumes (kidney beans, mixed beans, baked beans, lentils, chickpeas, black beans, pinto beans, butter beans, broad beans, chana dal)

VEGETABLES

- Peas
- Sweet corn
- Sweet potato
- Canned new potatoes
- Carrots

Other canned vegetables such as tomatoes, asparagus, peas and mushrooms are handy to boost the vegetable content of a meal. Other convenient products are:

- Tomato paste
- Tomato puree
- Bottled tomato pasta sauces
- Frozen vegetables

FRUITS

- Cherries
- Grapefruit
- Pears
- Apples

- Plums
- Peaches
- Oranges
- Grapes
- Kiwi
- Dried fruits, such as dried apricots, fruit medley, raisins and prunes
- Canned peaches, pears, apple as a useful standby
- Frozen berries and melon balls

DAIRY FOODS

- Shelf-stable skim milk or skim milk powder—easy to use in cooking
- Canned evaporated skim milk
- Cook 'n' Serve Sugar-Free Pudding and Pie Filling
- Skim or 1% milk
- Nonfat plain yogurt
- Light fruited yogurt
- Low fat ice cream
- Frozen low fat yogurt, sorbet, gelato
- Eggs

Cheese
- Low fat processed slices
- Reduced fat Swiss (such as Jarlsberg Light)
- Grated parmesan
- 1% or 2% cottage or part skim ricotta cheese

USEFUL FLAVORINGS, SAUCES AND DRESSINGS

- Spices—curry powder, cumin, turmeric, mustard, etc.

- Herbs—oregano, basil, thyme, etc.
- Bottled minced ginger, chili and garlic
- Sauces (such as soy, chili, oyster, hoisin, teriyaki, Worcestershire)
- Bouillon
- Low fat salad dressings

HYPOGLYCEMIA:
THE EXCEPTION TO THE LOW G.I. RULE

If you take insulin or pills to treat diabetes, your blood sugar level may sometimes fall below 70 milligrams per deciliter, which is the lower end of the normal range. When this happens you might feel hungry, shaky or sweaty and be unable to think clearly. This is called low blood sugar or "hypoglycemia."

Hypoglycemia is a potentially dangerous situation and must be treated right away by eating some carbohydrate food. In this case you should pick a carbohydrate with a high glycemic index because you need to increase your blood sugar quickly. Jelly beans (G.I. 80) are a good choice. If you are not due for your next meal or snack, you should also have some low G.I. carbohydrate (an apple, for example), to keep your blood sugar from falling again until you next eat.

■

GLUCOSE TABLETS OR JELLY BEANS ARE GOOD CHOICES FOR TREATING LOW BLOOD SUGAR.

■

Chapter 12

LOW G.I. EATING MADE EASY

BREAKFAST BASICS

LIGHT LUNCH IDEAS

A food is not good or bad on the basis of its glycemic index. Eating the low G.I. way means eating a variety of foods—possibly a wider variety than you are already eating.

Usually we eat a combination of carbohydrate foods, such as sandwiches and fruit, pasta and bread, cereal and toast, potatoes and corn. The glycemic index of a meal consisting of a mixture of carbohydrate foods is a weighted average of the glycemic index of the carbohydrate foods. The weighting is based on the proportion of the total carbohydrate contributed by each food. Studies show that when a food with a high glycemic index is combined with a food with a low glycemic index the complete meal has an intermediate glycemic index.

G.I. RANGES

Low G.I. Foods	below 55
Intermediate G.I. Foods	between 55 and 70
High G.I. Foods	more than 70

As with calories, the G.I. value is not precise. The glycemic index gives you a guide to help you lower the glycemic index of your day, and just one simple change can make a big difference. Look at the following ideas for the meals in your day and see how you could lower the glycemic index of your diet.

ARE YOU REALLY CHOOSING LOW FAT?

There's a trick to food labels that it is worth being aware of when shopping for low fat foods. These food labeling specifications guidelines were enacted by the United States Department of Agriculture (USDA) in 1994:

Free: Contains a tiny or insignificant amount of fat, cholesterol, sodium, sugar or calories; less than 0.5 grams (g) of fat per serving.

Low fat: Contains no more than 3 g of fat per serving.

Reduced/Less/Fewer: These diet products must contain 25 percent less of a nutrient or calories than the regular product.

Light/Lite: These diet products contain one-third fewer calories than, or half the fat of, the original product.

Lean: Meats claiming this contain less than 10 g of fat, 4 g of saturated fat, and 95 milligrams (mg) of cholesterol per serving.

Extra lean: These meats have less than 5 g of fat, 2 g of saturated fat, 95 mg of cholesterol.

BREAKFAST BASICS

1. Start with some fruit or juice

Fruit contributes fiber and, more important, vitamin C, which helps your body absorb iron. The lowest G.I. fruits and juices are:

Cherries	22	Dried apricots	31	Grapes	43
Plums	24	Apples	36	Oranges	43
Grapefruit	25	Pears	36	Pineapple juice	46
Peaches	28	Apple juice	41	Grapefruit juice	48

2. Try some breakfast cereal

Cereals are important as a source of fiber, vitamin B and iron. When choosing processed breakfast cereals, look for those with a high fiber content. Some of the lowest G.I cereals are:

Rice bran	19
Muesli, toasted	43
Bran Buds with Psyllium™	45
Oatmeal (made with water), cooked	49 (av)
Oat bran, Breakfast Cereal, Quaker Oats	50
All-Bran with extra fiber™	51
Frosted Flakes™	55
Oat bran, raw	55
Muesli, natural	56

3. Add milk or yogurt

Low fat milks and yogurts can make a valuable contribution to your daily calcium intake when you include them at breakfast. All have a low glycemic index, and lower fat varieties have just as much, or more, calcium as whole milk.

■ ■ ■

4. Then add some bread or toast, if you'd like
The lowest G.I. breads are:

Chapati (baisen)	27
Banana bread	47
Natural Ovens 100% Whole Grain	51
Whole grain pumpernickel	51
Sourdough	52
100% stoneground whole wheat	53
Whole wheat pita	57
Arnold's rye	57
Natural Ovens Hunger Filler	59
Natural Ovens Natural Wheat	59
Natural Ovens Happiness	63

---

10 QUICK, LOW FAT, LOW G.I. BREAKFAST IDEAS

- Spread raisin toast with low fat cream cheese and top with sliced apple or peach.
- Toast a slice of 100% stoneground whole wheat bread, on it melt 1 ounce slice of low fat cheese.
- Sprinkle oatmeal with raisins and brown sugar.
- Enjoy a low fat milkshake.
- Spoon a sliced peach and ¼ cup of raspberries through a container of light yogurt.
- Top a bowl of All-Bran and skim milk with canned pear slices.
- Spread 1 tablespoon natural peanut butter and 2 teaspoons spreadable fruit on 2 slices of sourdough toast.
- Team a cup of Quaker Oats oat bran and skim milk with a glass of fresh orange juice.
- Toast a whole wheat pita and top with 2 tablespoons cottage cheese or light ricotta.

■ Enjoy a steaming hot chocolate (made with skim milk) with sourdough toast and apple butter.

LIGHT LUNCH IDEAS

Include foods such as:

Bread roll	Pasta salad	Sweet corn
Grain bread	Pea soup	Tabouli
Lentil soup	Pita bread	Toast
Minestrone	Raisin toast	Vegetarian chili
Mixed bean salad	Ravioli	
Noodles	Rice salad	
Pasta	Steamed rice	

1. Base your light meals on carbohydrate

2. You might add a little meat, cheese, egg, or fish
Remember: the quantity of carbohydrate should be high, the add-ons should be accents. Here are some ideas:

- Bacon, just a sprinkle of lean, chopped
- Cheddar cheese, a couple of small cubes
- Chicken breast, about ¼ cup, chopped, boiled, grilled, baked
- Egg, hard boiled and quartered
- Ham, a thin slice
- Parmesan, a sprinkling of grated
- Pastrami, a lean slice
- Paté, a smearing
- Roast beef, a lean slice
- Sardines, a couple with lemon
- Smoked oysters, 3 to 4
- Smoked salmon, a slice

- Tuna, a tiny tin in water
- Turkey breast, a thin slice
- Yogurt, a small container of low fat

3. Fill it out with vegetables
Here are some suggestions:

Baby beets, whole	Spinach
Cabbage, shredded	Olives (up to 5)
Pepper strips	Salad greens
Carrot, grated	Shallots or onions, sliced
Cauliflower florets	Snow peas
Celery sticks	Sprouts
Cherry, grape or plum tomatoes	Sun dried tomatoes
Cucumber	

4. And round it off with fruit

---

10 LOW G.I. LUNCHES ON THE GO

1. Spread a pita with hummus, then fill with tabouli.
2. Cook a bowl of pasta, mix with pesto or chopped fresh herbs, sun dried tomatoes and part skim ricotta.
3. Put your favorite sandwich filling on whole grain pumpernickel bread (grill the sandwich if you'd like).
4. Melt cheese over tomato on slices of 100% stoneground whole wheat bread.
5. Pour 8 ozs. light yogurt over 1½ cups of fresh fruit salad.
6. Mix a green salad with some bean salad, add 2 to 4 Ryvita™ crispbread crackers.
7. Team a bowl of chunky vegetable soup, thick with barley, beans and macaroni with a piece of fruit.
8. Enjoy a lentil or veggie burger with salsa and grilled vegetables and salad on a whole wheat sandwich bun.

9. Try some smoked salmon on pumpernickel with a slice of avocado.
10. Mix up a banana smoothie and couple it with a high fiber apple muffin.

_____

Chapter 13

MASTERING LOW G.I. MEALS

ON THE MENU:

CARBOHYDRATE

VEGETABLES

PROTEIN

FAT

DESSERT

*J*ust one of the advantages of a low G.I. diet is the tremendous variety of foods it offers. You can eat just about anything you want—including dessert! Let the ideas below jump-start your menu-planning creativity.

1. FIRST CHOOSE THE CARBOHYDRATE

Which will it be? A new or sweet potato, Basmati or Uncle Ben's Converted Rice, a type of pasta, a grain, such as cracked wheat or barley, chickpeas, lentils and beans or a combination? Could you add some bread or corn?

2. ADD VEGETABLES—AND LOTS OF THEM

Fresh, frozen or canned—the more the merrier.

Artichokes	Eggplant	Radishes
Asparagus	Fennel	Salad greens
Beans	Leeks	Squash
Bok choy	Mushrooms	Tomatoes
Brussels sprouts	Okra	Zucchini
Cabbage	Onions	
Carrots	Peas	
Cauliflower	Pea pods	
Celery	Peppers	

3. NOW, JUST A LITTLE PROTEIN FOR FLAVOR AND TEXTURE

Remember, you don't need much—some slivers of beef to stir fry, a sprinkle of tasty cheese, strips of ham, a dollop of ricotta, a tender chicken breast, slices of salmon, a couple of eggs, a handful of nuts, or use the protein found in your grains and legumes.

4. THINK TWICE ABOUT USING ANY FAT

Check that you are using a healthy type (monounsaturated or polyunsaturated).

■ ■ ■

10 LOW G.I. DINNER IDEAS

- Team Spaghetti Bolognese with a green salad.
- Wrap a fish fillet dressed with herbs and lemon, or tomato and onion, in foil and bake. Serve with a heavy grain bread roll, mixed vegetables or salad.
- Stirfry chicken, meat or fish with mixed green vegetables. Serve with Basmati rice or Chinese noodles.
- Grill a steak and serve with a trio of low G.I. starchy vegetables—new potato, sweet corn and peas.
- Make a quick and easy omelette filled with vegetables, beans, ham, cheese or salsa and serve with rice.
- Cook spinach and ricotta tortellini, team up with fresh garden vegetables and top with a tomato pasta sauce.
- Create a one-pot chicken casserole with your favorite vegetables, chunks of new potatoes and barley.
- Make a lasagna—layer it with vegetables and some beans or beef and serve it with salad.
- Buy a barbecued chicken, steam sweet ears of corn and toss a salad together. Add pumpernickel bread.
- Wrap beef or chicken and beans in a soft tortilla. Heat in the oven or microwave. Top with salsa and serve with a salad. *Jennie's tip for those of you pressed for time*: Buy one take-out meal, split it with your partner. Round out the meal with home-cooked low G.I. rice or pasta plus loads of vegetables.

DESSERTS: A LOW G.I. FINISH

Although often overlooked, desserts can make a valuable contribution to your daily calcium and vitamin C intake when they are based on low fat dairy foods and fruits. Recipes incorporating fruit for sweetness will have more fiber and lower G.I. values than recipes with sugar. What's more, desserts are usually carbohydrate rich which means they help top-up our satiety center, signifying the completion of eating and reducing the tendency for late night nibbles.

If you haven't time to prepare a dessert, why not simply serve a bowl of fruits in season or a fruit platter with ricotta cheese? Remember, temperate climate fruits such as apples, pears and stone fruits tend to have the lowest G.I. values.

Apples	Kiwi
Apricots	Lychees
Bananas	Mandarins
Blueberries	Mangoes
Cantaloupe	Nectarines
Cherries	Oranges
Dates	Papaya
Figs	Peaches
Grapefruit	Pears
Grapes	Persimmons
Honeydew melon	Pineapple
Plums	Prunes
Quinces	Raspberries
Rhubarb	Star fruit
Strawberries	Watermelon

10 QUICK AND EASY LOW G.I. DESSERTS

- Try some low fat ice cream and strawberries.
- Bake a whole apple stuffed with dried fruit.
- Mix together a fruit salad with light yogurt.
- Make a fruit crisp: top cooked fruit with a crumbled mixture of toasted muesli, wheat flakes, a little melted butter (polyunsaturated or monounsaturated) and honey.
- Slice a firm banana into some low fat pudding.
- Top unsweetened canned fruit (peaches or pears) with low fat ice cream or low fat frozen yogurt.
- Wrap sliced apples, raisins, currants and spice, in a sheet

  of filo pastry (brushed with milk, not fat) and bake as a strudel.
- Make a winter fruit salad with segments of citrus fruits plus raisins soaked in orange juice, honey and brandy.
- Team unsweetened canned fruit with a dollop of plain yogurt and a sprinkle of toasted muesli.
- Enjoy a mousse made with 1% milk or yogurt and set with fruit.

■

A RULE OF THUMB:
HIGH G.I. FOOD + LOW G.I. FOOD
= INTERMEDIATE G.I. MEAL

■

Chapter 14

A WEEK OF LOW G.I. MENUS

CALORIES

FAT

CARBOHYDRATE

FIBER

MENUS

5 LITTLE TIPS THAT MAKE A BIG DIFFERENCE

This week of menus shows you how to eat a healthy, low G.I. diet. Use the menus for ideas to make sure you eat low fat, high carbohydrate, low G.I. meals every day.

We have included between-meal snacks in most of the menus as people who take medication (including insulin) to help control their diabetes generally need them. While not everyone with diabetes has to eat between meals, snacks can be a normal part of a healthy diet.

We have analyzed each menu to estimate its calories and the amount of fat, carbohydrate and fiber. We have also calculated the G.I. values. By emphasizing low G.I. foods, we have created menus with predicted low G.I. numbers, that is, below 55. Here are some points to consider.

1. CALORIES

Calories are a measure of the total amount of energy available from a food. Each day you require a certain amount of calories to fuel your body. The younger and more active you are the more energy you need. If you want to lose weight, you may need to reduce your calorie intake. The calorie levels of these menus are reasonably low and represent a minimum requirement for most people.

2. FAT

People with diabetes are advised to eat a low fat diet. The menus are examples of low fat meals if you use skim milk and minimal amounts of butter and other fats and oils when preparing them. If you are trying to lose weight, aim for a fat intake of 30 to 50 grams (g) per day. Remember, such low fat diets are not recommended for young children.

3. CARBOHYDRATE

These menus are all high in carbohydrate, deriving about half the total calories from that nutrient. For a small eater, this represents about 150 to 200 g of carbohydrate per day. The more active you are the more carbohydrate you need. Note that 150 to 200 g carbohydrate equates to 10 to 15 carbohydrate exchanges (for people who use that system).

4. FIBER

Guidelines suggest you need at least 30 g of fiber each day. This is often difficult to achieve on a low calorie intake without eating a high fiber cereal every morning. The fiber content of these menus varies from 20 to 40 g per day, giving a daily average of 30 g.

5 LITTLE TIPS THAT MAKE A BIG DIFFERENCE

- Think of carbohydrate foods as the number one priority in your meals.
- Change a dietary staple (such as bread) to a low G.I. staple to lower the overall glycemic index of your meals that day.
- Get in touch with your true appetite and use it to guide the amount of food you eat. Low fat, high fiber, low G.I. foods fill you up best.
- Try to eat at least two low G.I. meals each day.
- Mix high G.I. foods with low G.I. foods in your meals—the combination will give an overall intermediate glycemic index.

DID YOU KNOW?

You're less likely to overeat if you eat high carbohydrate, low G.I. foods. They'll make you feel full (or even too full) and satisfied before you've eaten more than your body needs.

MONDAY

G.I.:	47
TOTAL ENERGY:	1531 cal.
FAT:	31 g
CARBOHYDRATE:	231 g
FIBER:	40 g

Breakfast: Cereal and toast
One-half cup Raisin Bran with ½ cup 1% milk, 1 slice of 100% stoneground whole wheat bread, toasted, with 1 tablespoon of light margarine and 1 teaspoon of spreadable fruit.

Morning snack:
An apple

Lunch: Tuna-topped open sandwich and salad
Combine ½ cup of canned tuna with a little onion, parsley and 1 tablespoon low fat mayonnaise. Pile it on top of sliced tomato on 2 slices of 100% stoneground whole wheat bread and team it with 1 cup of mixed bean salad and salad greens.

Afternoon snack:
One cup of grapes (3 ounces)

Dinner: Grilled steak and vegetables
Broil or barbecue a piece of sirloin steak (about 4 ounces raw weight), basting with a marinade if desired. Cook a 3 ounce new potato in its skin and serve with a small ear of corn, and 1 cup of steamed baby carrots.

Evening snack:
An 8 ounce container of light fruited yogurt

TUESDAY

G.I.:	44
TOTAL ENERGY:	1562 cal.
FAT:	38 g
CARBOHYDRATE:	221 g
FIBER:	28 g

Breakfast: Oatmeal
Cook ½ cup rolled oats with ½ cup water and ½ cup skim milk. Serve with a teaspoon of brown sugar or a tablespoon of raisins.

Morning snack:
An orange

Lunch: A sandwich on the run
Cheese and salad on whole wheat bread.

Afternoon snack:
An 8 ounce container of light yogurt

Dinner: Pasta and sauce
Top about 1½ cups cooked pasta with ¾ cup of tomato or Bolognese (meat) sauce and a sprinkle of grated Parmesan cheese. Include a large salad with fat free dressing and a glass of red wine if desired. For dessert, help yourself to a large baked apple sprinkled with cinnamon.

Evening snack:
A bunch of grapes

WEDNESDAY

G.I.:	44
TOTAL ENERGY:	1573 cal.
FAT:	41 g
CARBOHYDRATE:	218 g
FIBER:	36 g

Breakfast: Cereal, fruit and toast
One-half cup All Bran with ½ cup unsweetened canned peaches and ¾ cup skim milk, 1 slice of 100% stoneground whole wheat toast with ½ teaspoon natural peanut butter.

Morning snack:
Two oatmeal cookies and ¾ cup skim milk.

Lunch: A toasted sandwich
2 ounces ham and tomato on 2 slices toasted pumpernickel bread. Finish with an apple.

Afternoon snack:
An orange

Dinner: Stir fry and rice
Stir-fry flank steak strips (about 3½ ounces raw weight) and a combination of at least 1 cup vegetables (such as broccoli, zucchini, shallots, cabbage), adding 1 tablespoon peanut oil, soy sauce, ginger, garlic, etc. to flavor. Serve with a cup of boiled rice such as Basmati or Uncle Ben's Converted Rice.

Evening snack:
A juicy peach or other fresh fruit in season

THURSDAY

G.I.:	46
TOTAL ENERGY:	1464 cal.
FAT:	24 g
CARBOHYDRATE:	231 g
FIBER:	38 g

Breakfast: Muesli, fruit and yogurt
Two-thirds cup Swiss style muesli with 6 ounces light fruited yogurt and a fresh sliced pear.

Morning snack:
Two Ryvita with 1 tablespoon natural peanut butter

Lunch: A filled spud
Microwave a large 9 ounce stuffing potato in its skin. Slice off the top, scoop out the middle, mix the potato with 1 tablespoon each of cottage cheese, diced ham, reduced fat Cheddar cheese and a sprinkle of chopped scallions. Stuff this mixture into the potato skin and reheat.

Afternoon snack:
One cup low fat chocolate milk

Dinner: Mexican beef and beans
Fill a 2 ounce pita with ½ cup stir fried kidney beans and 3 ounces of beef strips. Top with shredded lettuce, diced tomato and a sprinkle of reduced fat Cheddar cheese.

Evening snack:
A large apple

FRIDAY

G.I.:	47
TOTAL ENERGY:	1690 cal.
FAT:	50 g
CARBOHYDRATE:	215 g
FIBER:	27 g

Breakfast: Egg, toast and orange juice
One egg, prepared as desired (use vegetable spray if cooking in a pan). Toast 2 slices of pumpernickel bread and spread with 1 tablespoon of light margarine. Include 4 ounce glass of orange juice.

Morning snack:
Four Social Tea biscuits with tea or coffee

Lunch: A healthy wrap
Wrap ½ cup tabouli, 2½ ounce veggie burger (crumbled), 1 cup shredded lettuce, 1 small tomato, and 1 ounce low fat shredded cheese in a 2 ounce soft tortilla.

Afternoon snack:
A couple of kiwi

Dinner: Pasta with chicken, sautéed mushrooms and scallions
Gently sauté 1 cup mushrooms with ½ cup scallions, garlic and fresh parsley. When the vegetables are cooked, toss in 3 ounces diced cooked chicken breast. Serve over 1½ cups steaming fettucine. Accompany with 1 cup of sliced tomato and oregano salad mixed with fat free Italian dressing.

Evening snack:
A slice of raisin toast spread with 1 tablespoon light cream cheese

SATURDAY

G.I.:	48
TOTAL ENERGY:	1496 cal.
FAT:	28 g
CARBOHYDRATE:	225 g
FIBER:	25 g

Breakfast: Banana smoothie and graham crackers
Whip up a small, 5 ounce banana, 4 ounces light yogurt, 4 ounces skim milk and 1 tablespoon honey in a blender to make a quick liquid breakfast. Serve with 4 graham cracker squares. Save any leftovers for a morning snack.

Lunch: Grilled cheese and tomato
Cover 2 slices of sourdough bread each with 2 or 3 thin tomato slices and 1 ounce low fat Cheddar cheese. Heat in toaster oven or microwave until the cheese melts. Finish off with an orange.

Afternoon snack:
A crisp apple

Dinner: Roast pork with trimmings
Serve lean roast pork (about 4 ounces) with ½ cup natural apple sauce, a medium-sized dry roasted sweet potato, 1 cup steamed zucchini and green salad. Add a glass of wine if you like and top the meal off with 8 ounces light vanilla or lemon yogurt sprinkled with ½ cup diced mango.

SUNDAY

G.I.:	50
TOTAL ENERGY:	1439 cal.
FAT:	27 g
CARBOHYDRATE:	204 g
FIBER:	25 g

Breakfast: Toast and hot chocolate

Spread 2 slices of 100% stoneground whole wheat toast with 2 tablespoons part-skim ricotta cheese. Serve with hot chocolate made with skim milk. Add 1 medium grapefruit.

Morning snack:

A low fat granola bar

Lunch: Soup and salad

Heat up 1 cup tomato soup. Prepare a large tossed salad with mixed fresh vegetables and 2 ounces grilled chicken breast; top with your favorite low calorie fat free dressing.

Afternoon snack: An ice cream cone

One scoop (½ cup) low fat ice cream

Dinner: Fish, fries and salad

Cut a 6 ounce new potato into strips, spray with cooking oil, spread on baking tray and bake in a very hot oven until browned. Wrap a piece of fresh fish (about 5 ounces) in foil with fresh or dried herbs, lemon juice and/or white wine. Bake it for the last 10 to 15 minutes with the potatoes. Toss together lettuce, cucumber and shallots with vinegar and 1 teaspoon olive oil.

Evening snack:

A bunch of grapes or other fruit

Chapter 15

G.I. SUCCESS STORIES

*J*ust in case you're not yet convinced that a low G.I. diet can help you manage your diabetes, dietitian Johanna Burani, M.S., R.D., C.D.E., offers these three real-life examples from her own practice. Many of Johanna's patients have controlled their diabetes, lost weight and gained overall better health by choosing a low G.I. way of life.

MARGARINE: FRIEND OR FOE?

You'll notice that in some of the meals below, Johanna suggests using light margarine. As you may know, many margarines are sources of trans fats, which can raise cholesterol levels and have been implicated in increased risk of heart attacks and possibly even breast cancer. Luckily, not all margarine is created equal! Some products now on store shelves clearly boast that they are trans-fat free (look for those). Here are some other guidelines Johanna suggests you follow to avoid these unhealthy fats:

- Buy margarine by the tub, not the stick
- Look for "light," "low fat," "nonfat" or "fat free" on the label
- Make sure the first ingredient says "liquid," such as "liquid corn oil" or "liquid safflower oil"

CASE STUDY #1: GESTATIONAL DIABETES
"Marianne"

Age: 30
Height: 5'6"
Weight: 198 pounds, pre-pregnancy (clinically defined as "morbidly obese")

Background:
Married with a three-year-old daughter, Marianne is a stay-at-home mom. She doesn't smoke or drink alcohol, and for exercise, she walks and plays with her daughter. During the third trimester of her last pregnancy, Marianne was diagnosed with pre-eclampsia (a toxemia accompanied by high blood pressure, water retention and protein in the urine). Her last child was born two weeks early by C-section.

This pregnancy, Marianne suffers from gestational diabetes, which was diagnosed in her seventh month of pregnancy. She takes no medications other than prenatal vitamins.

■ ■ ■

Marianne's "before" diet:
Breakfast: Two cups Team cereal, 4 ozs. skim milk, 4 ozs. orange juice
Snack: Two cups watermelon
Lunch: Bowl of chicken noodle soup, 6 saltines, 1 piece of string cheese, butterscotch candy, 1 cup unsweetened canned peaches, water
Snack: Two cups watermelon
Dinner: Large baked potato with sour cream, small baked chicken cutlet, sliced cucumber, water
Late night snack: One-half bag popcorn, water

MARIANNE'S "BEFORE"
NUTRITIONAL ANALYSIS:

Calories: 1400
Carbohydrate: 237 g (70%)
Protein: 59 g (17%)
Fat: 19 g (13%)
G.I.: 73

Johanna's nutritional assessment:
Marianne is grossly underconsuming in all food categories except starches. Her caloric intake is meeting only about two-thirds of her current needs. She should try to eliminate all processed foods high in sodium (such as canned soups) and should increase her dairy foods to at least 24 ounces of milk or the equivalent.

Along with increasing her milk intake, Marianne needs to increase her protein sources by adding 6 ounces of high quality proteins (poultry, fish, eggs, meats, and so on) proportioned throughout the day (three meals plus a bedtime snack). She also needs to increase her vegetable portions at both lunch and dinner, and include condiments to help provide the required 35 percent calories from fat.

G.I.-specific counseling:

Marianne should try to replace her current cereal and cracker choices with whole grain options, substitute high G.I. fruits (watermelon and pineapple) with low G.I. options (apples, cherries, grapefruit, peaches, and so on) and replace the baked potato with noodles or long grain rice. Those changes will help produce lower G.I. meals that will help regulate Marianne's blood sugar levels for the duration of her pregnancy.

Marianne's new, low G.I. menu:

Breakfast: Two slices 100% stoneground whole wheat toast, 2 pats of butter, 1 egg, 8 ozs. 2% milk
Snack: Small bran muffin, 8 ozs. low fat plain yogurt
Lunch: Roast beef (2 ozs.) sandwich with 2 slices sourdough bread, a tomato and cucumber salad dressed with 2 tablespoons salad dressing, 4 ozs. unsweetened canned peaches, water
Snack: One oz. potato chips, 4 ozs. apple juice
Dinner: One cup spaghetti with marinara sauce, a 2 oz. meatball, 1 cup asparagus tips, 2 pats butter, medium orange, water
Snack: An 8 oz. glass of 2% milk, 3 graham cracker squares and 1 tablespoon natural peanut butter (no added salt)

MARIANNE'S "AFTER" NUTRITIONAL ANALYSIS:

Calories: 2100
Carbohydrate: 236 g (45%)

Protein: 101 g (19%)
Fat: 84 g (36%)
G.I.: 46

Marianne's winning results:
Marianne delivered a full-term healthy baby girl by
C-section and gained a total of 17 pounds throughout her pregnancy. Her blood sugar remained within
the normal ranges without the need of exogenous
insulin and her blood pressure was also stable and
within normal ranges without medication.

Marianne's comments:
"I'm so relieved the pregnancy turned out so well. I
was worried about the gestational diabetes but we
were able to control it with my diet. That's why I'm
anxious to get on a permanent meal plan—it's the
best way I can think of to prevent my getting type 2
diabetes."

CASE STUDY #2: TYPE 2 DIABETES
"Tony"

Age: 60
Height: 5'3"
Weight: 190 pounds (clinically defined as "morbidly obese")

Background:
Tony is married, works as a full-time school adminis-
trator and doesn't smoke or drink alcohol. For exercise, he walks for at least one hour every day. Tony
has just been diagnosed with type 2 diabetes and was
sent to Johanna to see whether dietary changes could

control his diabetes so medication wouldn't be necessary. Tony also suffers from borderline high blood pressure.

Tony's "before" diet:
Breakfast: A small pastry or muffin, and coffee throughout the morning
Lunch: He usually skips lunch on work days; an occasional business lunch would consist of tuna steak, roll, cole slaw, French fries and diet Coke
Dinner: Four hot dogs, tossed salad dressed with oil, vinegar and bacon bits, small piece of Italian bread, diet iced tea and coffee
Snack: Glass of skim milk

TONY'S "BEFORE" NUTRITIONAL ANALYSIS:

Calories: 2700
Carbohydrate: 149 g (22%)
Protein: 154 g (23%)
Fat: 163 g (55%)
G.I.: 67

Johanna's nutritional assessment:
The best strategy to address Tony's multiple medical problems (diabetes, hypertension, obesity) all at once is to correct his diet. He would need to decrease his fat and sodium intake and increase his carbohydrates in the form of fruits, vegetables and whole grains, and eat minimally processed foods. He should consume his daily calories in three meals and one or two snacks. He should attempt to drink 64 ozs. of water throughout the day.

Tony needs to reduce his fat from his current 55 percent of calories to less than 30 percent. He needs to include three or four servings of fruit with meals and snacks. He needs to follow some brown bag lunch guidelines and identify the proper portion sizes for evening entrees, with an emphasis on low fat choices.

G.I.-specific counseling:
Although Tony's carbohydrate foods fall into the "intermediate G.I." category, those foods contribute a paltry 22 percent of his caloric intake on an average day. His high fat foods are making him feel full. He'll still feel full if he replaces these calorically dense foods with low G.I. carbohydrates, but will be consuming less than half the calories.

Tony's new, low G.I. menu:
Breakfast: Three-quarters cup Raisin Bran, 8 ozs. skim milk, coffee, ½ cup unsweetened canned peaches

Lunch: Roasted turkey breast (2 ozs.) sandwich on 2 slices multigrain bread, 1 cup cantaloupe, water or decaf diet beverage

Snack: An 8 oz. container of light yogurt

Dinner: One and a half cups fettucine with marinara sauce, 3 oz. pan fried breaded pork cutlet, 1 tablespoon olive oil, 1 cup spinach, 4 ozs. natural applesauce, water

Snack: An 8 oz. cup of skim milk, oatmeal cookie

TONY'S "AFTER" NUTRITIONAL ANALYSIS:

Calories: 1500
Carbohydrate: 211 g (55%)

Protein: 86 g (22%)
Fat: 39 g (23%)
G.I.: 43

Tony's winning results:
Tony reached his initial goal weight of 160 pounds after five months of eating low G.I. meals and snacks. He takes no medications for either diabetes or high blood pressure. At my recommendation, he will maintain this weight for the next two to three months, at which time we'll design a new meal plan and exercise program to promote further gradual loss of another 10 to 20 pounds.

Tony's comments:
"I've never felt better in my life!"

CASE STUDY #3: TYPE 1 DIABETES
"Joyce"

Age: 64
Height: 5'6"
Weight: 227 pounds (clinically defined as "morbidly obese")

Background:
Joyce is an unmarried professional full-time cook. She neither smokes nor drinks alcohol and walks every day for 20 minutes (when she isn't feeling sick). Joyce has a number of health problems: She suffers from high blood pressure and is taking multiple medications to control her diabetes. She also injects insulin twice a day (total of 111 units) and takes one oral agent as well. Her blood sugar numbers range above 330, indi-

cating poor control. Joyce's cholesterol is also high, though she takes no medications for that condition.

Joyce's "before" diet:
Breakfast: Fried egg, 2 slices of whole wheat toast with margarine, coffee with 2% milk
Snack: An 8 oz. glass of apple juice
Lunch: Baked fish, ½ cup hash brown potatoes, creamed spinach, apple, water
Dinner: Two slices of pizza, a handful of chips, 2 bologna slices, apple, water
Late night snack: Handful of pretzel nuggets

JOYCE'S "BEFORE" NUTRITIONAL ANALYSIS:

Calories: 2200
Carbohydrate: 235 g (42%)
Protein: 87 g (15%)
Fat: 106 g (43%)
G.I.: 56

Johanna's nutritional assessment:
Because Joyce is morbidly obese and carries her excess fat abdominally, her body is resistant to insulin; even though she is taking large doses, her sugar control remained unsatisfactory. Joyce will need to reduce her caloric intake (specifically her fat calories) and balance her diet with more vegetables and low fat dairy foods.

G.I.-specific counseling:
Joyce's carbohydrate choices consist predominantly of low or intermediate G.I. foods, which is a good

start. By balancing her meals and snacks with more whole grains, vegetables and low fat dairy foods, and reducing her fat calories, she will start losing some weight and become less insulin-resistant, without feeling hungry. Her low G.I. food choices will simultaneously help lower her weight, blood sugars, blood pressure and cholesterol levels and give her more energy.

Joyce's new, low G.I. menu:
Breakfast: One and one-third cups of All Bran with extra fiber, 8 ozs. of skim milk, small apple
Lunch: One cup noodles, 4 ozs. broiled chicken breast, 1 cup green beans, tossed salad dressed with 1 teaspoon olive oil and vinegar, 3 ozs. cherries, water
Dinner: Two-thirds cup Uncle Ben's Converted Rice, 4 ozs. lemon sole, 1 cup steamed broccoli and cauliflower florets, 1 tablespoon light margarine, 1 cup grapes, water
Snack: Eight graham cracker squares and 8 ozs. light yogurt

JOYCE'S "AFTER" NUTRITIONAL ANALYSIS:

Calories: 1700
Carbohydrate: 224 g (53%)
Protein: 90 g (21%)
Fat: 47 g (26%)
G.I.: 43

Joyce's winning results:
In the past six years, Joyce has lost 47 pounds, and has been able to maintain a weight of 180. Her blood

pressure and cholesterol levels have normalized. She is taking one insulin injection a day, having reduced her insulin requirement by 85 percent. Her blood sugars are all within the normal range.

Joyce's comments:
"It's so nice to have energy again. And I have more time on my hands now to work on my hobbies, since I go to the doctor less often."

Chapter 16

THE LOW G.I. CHECKLIST

BREAKFAST CEREALS

VEGETABLES

BREADS

COOKIES AND CAKES

JUICES

SNACK FOODS

CEREAL GRAINS AND PASTA

DAIRY FOODS

LEGUMES

FRUIT

LOW G.I. SUBSTITUTES

*G*oing grocery shopping? Bring this list with you. It will help you choose low G.I. foods quickly and easily.

BREAKFAST CEREALS

Rice bran	19
Muesli, toasted	43
Bran Buds with Psyllium™	45
Oatmeal (made with water), cooked	49 (av)
Oat bran	50
All-Bran with extra fiber™	51
Frosted Flakes™	55

Oat bran, raw	55
Muesli, natural	56

VEGETABLES

Peas	48
Yam	51
Sweet potato	54
Corn	55
New potato, canned	61

BREADS

Chapati (baisen)	27
Banana bread	47
Natural Ovens 100% Whole Grain Bread	51
Whole grain pumpernickel	51
Sourdough	52
100% stoneground whole wheat	53
Whole wheat pita bread	57
Arnold's rye	57
Natural Ovens Hunger Filler Bread	59
Natural Ovens Natural Wheat Bread	59
Natural Ovens Happiness Bread	63

COOKIES AND CAKES

Apple cinnamon muffin, from mix*	44
Sponge cake	46
Banana bread*	47
Oatmeal cookie	55
Social Tea biscuits™	55

JUICES

Apple juice, unsweetened	40
Pineapple juice, unsweetened	46
Orange juice	46
Grapefruit juice	48

SNACK FOODS

Chocolate bar*	49
Potato chips*	54
Popcorn	55

CEREAL GRAINS AND PASTA

Pearled barley	25
Spaghetti	41
Macaroni	45
Uncle Ben's Converted™ Rice	44
Bulgur (cracked wheat)	48
Buckwheat	54
Brown rice	55
Long grain white rice	56

DAIRY FOODS

Yogurt, nonfat, artificially sweetened	14
Milk, whole	27
Milk, nonfat	32
Yogurt, nonfat, sweetened with sugar	33
Milk, chocolate flavored	34
Pudding, cooked	43
Ice cream, low fat	50

LEGUMES

Soy beans, boiled	18
Lentils, red, boiled	26
Kidney beans	27
Lentils, green and brown	30
Butter beans	31
Lima beans	32
Split peas	32
Chickpeas	33
Navy beans	38
Chickpeas, canned	42
Baked beans, canned	48
Kidney beans, canned	52

FRUIT

Cherries	22
Grapefruit	25
Peaches	28
Canned peaches, unsweetened	30
Dried apricots	31
Pears	38
Apples	38
Plums	39
Oranges	44
Grapes	46
Kiwi	52

Note: Canned legumes have higher G.I. values than the boiled varieties because the temperatures and pressures used in the canning process increase the digestibility of the starch. But, canned legumes are still an excellent low fat, high fiber, nutrient-rich low G.I. choice!

*Foods containing fat in excess of American Heart Association guidelines. Use these only once in a while and in small amounts.

LOW G.I. SUBSTITUTES

High G.I. Food	Low G.I. Alternative
Bread, whole wheat or white	Bread containing a lot of whole grains such as pumpernickel or 100% stoneground whole wheat
Processed breakfast cereal	Unrefined cereal such as old-fashioned oats. Check pages 111–123 for an A–Z list of more than 300 other foods and for processed cereals with low G.I. values (such as Bran Buds with Psyllium™)
Cookies and crackers	Cookies made with dried fruit and whole grains such as oats
Cakes and muffins	Look for those made with fruit, oats, whole grains
Tropical fruits	Temperate climate fruits such as bananas, apples, peaches and nectarines
Potato	Use new potatoes
Rice	Try Basmati, Uncle Ben's Converted™, brown or long grain rice

---

Chapter 17

YOUR QUESTIONS ANSWERED

WHICH IS BETTER:
A HIGH PROTEIN OR LOW G.I. DIET?
WHAT'S THE BEST DIET FOR DIABETES?
SHOULD YOU AVOID HIGH FAT FOODS?
DOES SUGAR CAUSE DIABETES?
AND MORE . . .

Could a high protein diet be harmful to a person with diabetes?

Yes. People with diabetes should avoid some high protein diets because eating large amounts of protein can bring on renal failure more quickly. (Renal failure is one possible complication of diabetes.) It's much healthier for people with diabetes to control their blood sugar by eating a low G.I. diet.

What are the other side effects of a high protein diet?

Some high protein diets are also harmful for elderly people and anyone with high blood pressure or diabetes. High protein, high fat diets can lead to high cholesterol, heart disease, and increase the risk of heart attack. These diets also lack fiber, which may lead to constipation. What's more, some high protein diets can reduce the intake of important vitamins, minerals, fiber and trace elements.

Why are diets that disregard widely accepted nutritional guidelines so fashionable right now?

Several best-selling books have been published promoting high protein diets and generating a lot of publicity. But the fact is: Diets that limit major food groups do not work over the long haul.

A high fat food may have a low glycemic index. Doesn't this give a falsely favorable impression of that food for people with diabetes?

Yes it does. The glycemic index of potato chips or French fries is lower than baked potatoes. The glycemic index of corn chips is lower than sweet corn. It is important not to base your food choices on the glycemic index alone; you need to consider the fat content of foods as well. Low fat eating helps control weight, especially for people with diabetes.

If a food has a high glycemic index, should someone with diabetes avoid it?

Not necessarily. A food isn't good or bad on the basis of its glycemic index. Eating the low G.I. way means eating a variety of foods—possibly a wider variety than you are already eating.

We generally tend to eat a combination of carbohydrate foods, such as sandwiches and fruit, pasta and bread, cereal and toast, potatoes and corn. The glycemic index of a meal consisting of a mixture of carbohydrate foods is a weighted average of the glycemic index of the carbohydrate foods. The weighting is based on the proportion of the total carbohydrate contributed by each food. Studies show that when a food with a high glycemic index is combined with a food with a low G.I. the complete meal has an intermediate glycemic index.

(Low G.I. foods have values at 55 or below; intermediate G.I. values are between 55 and 70, and high G.I. foods have values greater than 70.)

Some foods such as some breads and potatoes have high G.I. values (70 to 80). But, potatoes and bread can play a major role in a high carbohydrate and low fat diet. You only have to exchange about half the carbohydrate (from high to low glycemic index) to achieve improvements. So, there's plenty of room for bread and potatoes. Some breads and potatoes have a lower G.I. values than others. Choose these if your goal is to lower the glycemic index as much as possible.

Is it better to eat complex carbohydrate instead of simple sugars?

There are no big distinctions between sugars and starches in either nutritional terms or when it comes to G.I. values. Some sugars such as fructose or fruit sugar have a low glycemic index. Others, such as glucose, have a high glycemic index. The most common sugar in our diet, ordinary table sugar (sucrose), has a moderate glycemic index.

Starches can fall into both the high and low G.I. categories too, depending on the type of starch and what treatment it has received during cooking and processing. Most modern starchy foods (such as bread, potatoes and breakfast cereals), contain high G.I. carbohydrate.

What our research has shown is that you don't have to eliminate sugar completely from your diet. However, it is important to remember that sugar alone won't keep the engine running smoothly, so don't over-do it. A balanced diet contains a wide variety of foods.

Are naturally occurring sugars better than refined sugars?

Naturally occurring sugars are those found in foods such as fruit, vegetables and milk. Refined sugars are concentrated sources of sugar such as table sugar, honey or molasses.

The rate of digestion and absorption of naturally occurring sugars is no different, on average, from that of refined sugars. There is wide variation within both food groups, depending on the food. For example, the glycemic index of fruits ranges from 22 for cherries to 72 for watermelon. Similarly, among the foods containing refined sugars, some have low G.I. values, while others have high G.I. numbers. The glycemic index of sweetened yogurt is only 33, while each Life Savers candy has a glycemic index of 70 (the same as some breads).

Some nutritionists argue that naturally occurring sugars are better because they contain minerals and vitamins not found in refined sugar. However, recent studies which have analyzed high sugar and low sugar diets clearly show that the diets overall contain similar amounts of micronutrients. Studies have shown that people who eat moderate amounts of refined sugars have perfectly adequate micronutrient intakes.

Can people with diabetes eat as much sugar as they want?

Research shows that moderate consumption of refined sugar (about 8 teaspoons) a day doesn't compromise blood sugar control. This means you can choose foods which contain refined sugar or even use small amounts of table sugar. Try to spread your sugar budget over a variety of nutrient rich foods that sugar makes more palatable. Remember, sugar is concealed in many foods—a can of soft drink contains about 40 g sugar.

Most foods containing sugar do not raise blood sugar levels any more than most starchy foods. Golden Grahams (G.I. 71) contain 39 percent sugar while Rice Chex (G.I. 89) contain very little sugar. Many foods with large amounts of sugar have G.I. values close to 60—lower than white bread.

Sugar can be a source of enjoyment and help you limit your intake of high fat foods, but the blood sugar response to a food is hard to predict. Use the tables in this book and your own blood sugar monitoring as a guide.

Why should people with diabetes watch out for fatty foods?

With diabetes, being overweight and eating fatty foods prevents insulin from doing its job. When insulin can't work properly (or there isn't enough of it) blood sugar levels rise. Most type 2 (non-insulin-dependent) diabetes is associated with an excess of abdominal fat (a "pot belly").

Breaded or battered foods, French fries, fried rice, pastries or other such fatty foods are often the cause of elevated blood sugar. The high glycemic index of the potato, rice or flour tends to increase blood sugar levels, and the extra fat interferes with the action of insulin and makes it less effective in clearing sugar from the blood.

Some foods high in fat have a low glycemic index and may seem all right to eat because of this. The glycemic index is low because fat tends to slow the rate of stomach emptying (and therefore the rate at which foods are digested in the small intestine). Some high fat foods, therefore, tend to have lower G.I. values than their low fat equivalents (potato chips, 54 compared with a dry baked potato, 85). This doesn't make them better foods.

Has the glycemic index been tested in long-term studies?

At least 12 studies to date have looked at the glycemic index in the diet in relation to long-term diabetes control. Some of these studies have been five weeks long, others, including ours, up to three months. All but one showed a clear benefit in improving blood sugar levels. People with high blood lipids (cholesterol, triglycerides) showed improvements in this area as well.

The insulin response is important and the glycemic index does not tell us anything about this. Is there a correlation?

In general, studies have found an excellent correlation between the glycemic index of a food and its insulin response. Sometimes the insulin response is higher or lower than expected. The presence of more protein will increase the insulin response proportionately. A large amount of fat may reduce the glycemic response but not the insulin response. But we should be avoiding large amounts of fat.

Are G.I. values tested on healthy people valid for use in people with diabetes?

Yes, there are several studies which show a good correlation between values for the same foods obtained in healthy people and people with diabetes (type 1 and type 2). This is no surprise because the degree of glucose intolerance is allowed for in the calculation of the glycemic index.

One study gave carrots a glycemic index of 95. Does this mean that a person with diabetes should-n't eat carrots? What about other salad vegetables? And avocados?

The quantity of carrots that gives the 50 grams of carbohydrate portion (as used in standardized G.I. testing) is enormous because they contain only about 7 percent carbohydrate. In fact, a 25-gram carbohydrate portion of carrots (about ¾ pound) were tested. This is much greater than the amount you would normally eat (about 3½ ounces).

Even with a glycemic index of 95, a normal serving of carrots would contribute only a small amount to the rise in blood sugar. Carrots and other foods such as tomatoes, onions and salad vegetables that contain only a small amount of carbohydrate should be seen as "free" foods for people with diabetes.

Avocados are also insignificant sources of carbohydrate. Their glycemic index is effectively zero, and they therefore won't raise your blood sugar levels. They are rich in monounsaturated oils and many micronutrients, but unlike most other vegetables, they are also very high in fat and calories, so enjoy them in moderation.

If foods containing refined sugar have an intermediate glycemic index, does this mean that people with diabetes can eat as much sugar as they want?

Research has clearly shown that the glycemic index of refined sugar is the same in people who have diabetes and people who don't. Moderate consumption of sugar (which means 3 to 5 tablespoons of refined sugars a day) does not compromise blood sugar control. In fact, excluding sugar from the diet has important psychological consequences.

Sugar is not just empty calories, but a source of pleasure and reward and it helps to limit the intake of fatty foods and high G.I. carbohydrates.

Our advice is to spread your sugar budget over a variety of nutrient rich foods that become more palatable with the addition of sugar, such as yogurt, oatmeal and other breakfast cereals, jam on toast, milk drinks and fruit desserts.

What is chana dal?

Chana dal, the bean with the lowest glycemic index (G.I. 8), is a diet staple in India, but, as yet, is still little known in the United States. Scientifically, chana dal is the *desi* type of *Cicer arietinum*. The chana dal bean looks just like yellow split peas, but when cooked, it doesn't readily boil down to mush the way split peas do. It is more closely related to chickpeas (garbanzo beans), but chana dal is younger, smaller, sweeter, and has a much lower glycemic index. In fact, you can substitute chana dal for chickpeas in just about any recipe. Chana dal is generally available in Indian and Southeast Asian food stores, and as awareness of the value of eating low G.I. foods spreads, it is becoming more widely available. If you don't see it at your favorite food store, ask your local health food store or specialty grocer to carry it.

Bread and potatoes have high G.I. values (70 to 80). Does this mean a person with diabetes should avoid bread and potatoes?

Potatoes and bread can play a major role in a high carbohydrate and low fat diet, even if a secondary goal is to reduce the overall G.I. value. Only about half the carbohydrate has to be exchanged from high glycemic index to low glycemic index to achieve measurable improvements in diabetes control. So, there is still room for bread and potatoes. Of course, some types of bread and potatoes have lower G.I. values than others and these should be preferred if the goal is to lower the glycemic index as much as possible.

In the overall management of diabetes, the most important message is that the diet should be low in fat and high in carbohydrate. This will help people not only to lose weight, but to keep it off and improve their overall blood glucose and lipid control.

Chapter 18

LOW FAT, LOW G.I. RECIPE SECRETS

*A*s we have said constantly throughout this book, it is important to eat a high carbohydrate and low fat diet. The following practical tips that we have set out in an easy A to Z format will help you reduce the fat content of some of your favorite recipes while lowering their glycemic index.

Alcohol Although excessive alcohol consumption can be fattening, as an ingredient in a recipe, alcohol itself won't create a high calorie dish. Alcohol evaporates during cooking, so you lose the calories and are left with the flavor. A little wine in a sauce can give a delicious flavor, and sherry in an Asian style marinade is essential.

Bacon Bacon is a valuable ingredient in many dishes because of the flavor it offers. You can make a little bacon go a long way by trimming off all fat and chopping it finely. Lean ham is often a more economical and leaner way to go. In casseroles and soups, a ham bone imparts a fine flavor without much fat.

Cheese At around 30 percent fat (23 percent of this being saturated), cheese can contribute quite a lot of fat to a recipe. Although there are a number of fat-reduced cheeses available, many of these lose a lot in flavor for a small reduction in fat. It is worth comparing fat per ounce between brands to find the tastiest one with the lowest fat content. Alternatively, a sprinkle of a grated, very tasty cheese or Parmesan may do the job.

Part skim ricotta and cottage cheeses are lower fat alternatives to butter on a sandwich. It's worth trying some fresh part skim ricotta from a deli—you may find the texture and flavor more acceptable than that of the ricotta available in containers in the supermarket. Flavored cottage cheeses are ideal low fat toppings for crackers. Try ricotta in lasagna instead of a creamy white sauce.

Cream and sour cream Keep to very small amounts as these are high in saturated fat. Substitute nonfat sour cream, which tastes very similar to the full fat variety. A 16 ounce container of heavy cream can be poured into ice-cube trays and frozen providing small servings of cream easily when you need it. Adding one ice-cube block (1 oz.) of cream to a dish adds only 5½ grams of fat.

Dried beans, peas and lentils These are all low in fat and very nutritious. Incorporating them in a recipe, perhaps as a partial substitution for meat, will lower the fat content of the finished product. Canned beans, chickpeas and lentils are now widely available. They are very convenient to use and a great time saver. They are comparable in food value to the dried ones that you soak and cook yourself.

Eggs Be conscious of eggs in a recipe as they can add fat. Sometimes just the beaten egg white can be substituted for the whole egg, or use egg substitute.

Filo pastry Unlike most other pastry, filo (also known as phyllo) is low in fat. To keep it that way, brush between the sheets with skim milk instead of melted butter when you prepare it. Look for it in the freezer section of the supermarket with other prepared pastry and use it as a pie filling or a strudel wrap.

Grilling Grill or broil tender cuts of meat, chicken and fish rather than fry. Marinating first will add flavor, moisture and tenderness.

Health food stores Health food stores can be traps for the unwary. Check out the high fat ingredients, such as hydrogenated vegetable oil, nuts, coconut and palm kernel oil in the products such as granola bars, fruit bars and "healthy" cakes (even if made with whole wheat flour) that they stock on their shelves.

Ice cream A source of carbohydrate, calcium, riboflavin, retinol and protein. Low fat varieties have the lower glycemic index—definitely a nutritious and icy treat.

Jam A tablespoon of jam on toast contains far fewer calories than a pat of butter. So, enjoy your jam and give fat the flick!

Keep jars of minced garlic, chili or ginger in the refrigerator to spice up your cooking in an instant.

Lemon juice Try a fresh squeeze with ground black pepper on vegetables rather than a pat of butter. Lemon juice provides acidity that slows gastric emptying and lowers the glycemic index.

Milk Many people dislike skim milk, particularly when they taste it on its own or in their coffee! However, you can use skim milk in a recipe and no one will notice—and the fat savings is great. For convenience you might want to keep powdered skim milk in the pantry, which can be made up to the desired quantity when you need it. It will taste more like fresh milk if you mix the powder and water according to directions and refrigerate the milk overnight before using it. Ultra-pasteurized milk is handy in the cupboard, too.

Nuts They are valuable for their content of vitamin E, but they are also high in fat. To keep the fat content of a recipe low, the quantity of nuts has to be small.

Oil Most of our recipes call for no more than 2 teaspoons of oil. Any polyunsaturated or monounsaturated oil is suitable. Cooking spray or brushing oil lightly over the base of the pan is ideal. If you find the amount of oil insufficient, cover your pan, or add a few drops of water and use steam to cook the ingredients without burning. It is a good idea to invest in a nonstick frying pan if you don't have one!

Pasta A food to eat more of and a great source of carbohydrate and B vitamins. Fresh or dried, the preparation is easy. Just boil in water until just tender or "al dente," drain and top with a dollop of pesto, a tomato sauce or a sprinkle of Parmesan and pepper. There are many wonderful pasta cookbooks now available, and it's definitely worth investing in one to find all sorts of exciting ways to prepare this fabulous low G.I. food. Pasta may appear in your menu as a side dish to meat, as noodles in soup, as a meal in itself with vegetables or sauce or even as an ingredient in a dessert.

Questions Ask your dietitian for more recipe ideas. (See "For More Information" on page 125 to locate an R.D. near you.)

Reduce the fat content of ground beef by browning it in a nonstick pan, then placing the meat in a colander and pouring boiling water through it to wash away the fat. Return to the pan to continue cooking. It is a good idea to buy the better quality ground beef with less fat.

Stock If you are prepared to go to the effort of making your own stock—good for you! Prepare it in advance, refrigerate it then skim off the accumulated fat from the top. Prepared stock is available in long-life cartons and cans in the supermarket. Stock cubes are another alternative. Look for brands that have reduced salt.

To sauté Heat the pan first, brush with the recommended amount of oil (or less), add the food and cook, stirring lightly over a gentle heat.

Underlying the need for fat is a need for taste. Be creative with other flavorings.

Vinegar A vinaigrette dressing (1 tablespoon vinegar and 2 teaspoons of oil) with your salad can lower the blood sugar response to the whole meal by up to 30 percent. The best types of vinegars for this purpose are red or white wine vinegar. Another option: Use lemon juice.

Weighing What's the weight of the meat you're buying? Start noticing the weight that appears on the butcher's scales or package label and consider how many servings it will give you. With a food such as steak, that is basically all edible meat, 4 to 5 ounces per serving is sufficient. One pound is more than enough for 4 portions. Choose lean cuts of meat and trim away the fat before cooking or before you put it away. Alternate meat or chicken with fish once or twice a week.

Yogurt Yogurt is a valuable food in many ways. It is a good source of calcium, "friendly bacteria," protein and riboflavin, and unlike milk, is suitable for those people who are lactose intolerant. Low fat plain yogurt is a suitable substitute for sour cream. If using yogurt in a hot sauce or casserole, add it at the last minute and do not let it boil, or it will curdle. It is best if you can bring the yogurt to room temperature before adding to the hot dish. To do this, mix a small amount of yogurt with a little sauce from the dish, then stir this mixture back into the bulk of the sauce.

Zero fat Eating zero fat is unhealthy, so speak with a dietitian about how to get just the right amount you need. Our bodies need essential fatty acids that can't be synthesized and must be supplied in the diet. Fat does add flavor—use it to your advantage.

Chapter 19

HOW TO USE THE G.I. TABLES

The following table is an A to Z listing of the glycemic index values of commonly eaten foods in the United States and Canada. Approximately 300 different foods are listed, including some new values for foods tested only recently.

The glycemic index shown next to each food is the average for that food using glucose as the standard (i.e., glucose has a glycemic index of 100, with other foods rated accordingly). The average may represent the mean of 10 studies of that food worldwide or only two to four studies. In a few instances, American data are different from the rest of the world and we show that data rather than the average. Rice and oatmeal fall into this category.

To check on a food's glycemic index, simply look

for it by name in the alphabetic list. You may also find it under a food type—as fruit or cookies, for example.

Included in the tables is the carbohydrate (CHO) and fat content of a sample serving of the food. This is to help you keep track of the amount of fat and carbohydrate in your diet. The sample serving is not the recommended serving—it is just an example of a serving. The glycemic index does not depend on your serving size because it is a ranking of the glycemic effect of foods using carbohydrate-equivalent portion sizes. You can eat more of a low G.I. food or less of a high G.I. food and achieve the same blood sugar levels.

Remember when you are choosing foods, the glycemic index isn't the only thing to consider. In terms of your blood sugar levels you should also consider the amount of carbohydrate you are eating. For your overall health the fat, fiber and micronutrient content of your diet is also important. A dietitian can guide you further with good food choices; see "For More Information" on page 125 for advice on finding a dietitian.

■

FOR A SMALL EATER (1,500 CALORIES A DAY),
AIM FOR LESS THAN 50 G FAT A DAY
AND 188 G CARBOHYDRATE.

■

FOR A BIGGER EATER (2,500 CALORIES A DAY),
AIM FOR LESS THAN 80 G FAT A DAY
AND 313 G CARBOHYDRATE.

■

Chapter 20

THE GLYCEMIC INDEX TABLE

A–Z OF FOODS WITH GLYCEMIC INDEX, CARBOHYDRATE & FAT

Food	Glycemic Index	Fat (g per svg.)	CHO (g per svg.)
Agave nectar (90% fructose syrup), 1 tablespoon	11	0	16
All-Bran with extra fiber™, Kellogg's, breakfast cereal, ½ cup, 1 oz.	51 (av)	1	22
Angel food cake, ½₂ cake, 1 oz.	67	trace	17
Apple, 1 medium, 5 ozs.	38 (av)	0	18
Apple, dried, 1 oz.	29	0	24
Apple juice, unsweetened, 1 cup, 8 ozs.	40	0	29
Apple cinnamon muffin, from mix, 1 muffin	44	5	26
Apricots, fresh, 3 medium, 3 ozs.	57	0	12
canned, light syrup, 3 halves	64	0	14
dried, 5 halves	31	0	13
Apricot jam, no added sugar, 1 tablespoon	55	0	17
Apricot and honey muffin, low fat, from mix, 1 muffin	60	4	27
Bagel, 1 small, plain, 2.3 ozs.	72	1	38
Baked beans, ½ cup, 4 ozs.	48 (av)	1	24
Banana bread, 1 slice, 3 ozs.	47	7	46
Banana, raw, 1 medium, 5 ozs.	55 (av)	0	32
Banana, oat and honey muffin, low fat from mix, 1 muffin	65	4	27
Barley, pearled, boiled, ½ cup, 2.6 ozs.	25 (av)	0	22
Basmati white rice, boiled, 1 cup, 6 ozs.	58	0	50
Beets, canned, drained, ½ cup, 3 ozs.	64	0	5
Black bean soup, ½ cup, 4 ½ ozs.	64	2	19
Black beans, boiled, ¾ cup, 4.3 ozs.	30	1	31
Black bread, dark rye, 1 slice, 1.7 ozs.	76	1	18
Blackeyed peas, canned, ½ cup, 4 ozs.	42	1	16
Blueberry muffin, 1 muffin, 2 ozs.	59	4	27
Bran			
All-Bran with extra fiber™, Kellogg's, ½ cup, 1 oz.	51	1	20

Food	Glycemic Index	Fat (g per svg.)	CHO (g per svg.)
Bran Buds with Psyllium™, Kellogg's, ⅓ cup, 1 oz.	45	1	24
Bran Flakes, Post, ⅔ cup, 1 oz.	74	1	22
Multi-Bran Chex™, General Mills, 1 cup, 2.1 ozs.	58	15	49
Oat bran, 1 tablespoon	55	1	7
Oat bran muffin, 2 ozs.	60	4	28
Rice bran, 1 tablespoon	19	2	5
Breads			
Dark rye, Black bread, 1 slice, 1.7 ozs.	76	1	18
Dark rye, Schinkenbröt, 1 slice, 2 ozs.	86	1	22
French baguette, 1 oz.	95	1	15
Gluten-free bread, 1 slice	90	1	18
Hamburger bun, 1 prepacked bun, 1½ ozs.	61	2	22
Kaiser roll, 1, 2 ozs.	73	2	34
Light deli (American) rye, 1 slice, 1 oz.	68	1	16
Melba toast, 6 pieces, 1 oz.	70	2	23
Natural Ovens 100% Whole Grain, 1 slice, 1.2 ozs.	51	0	17
Natural Ovens Hunger Filler, 1 slice, 1.2 ozs.	59	0	16
Natural Ovens Natural Wheat, 1 slice, 1.2 ozs.	59	0	16
Natural Ovens Happiness, 1 slice, 1.1 oz.	63	0	15
Pita bread, whole wheat, 6½ inch loaf, 2 ozs.	57	2	35
Pumpernickel, whole grain, 1 slice, 1 oz.	51	1	15
Rye bread, 1 slice, 1 oz.	65	1	15
Sourdough, 1 slice, 1½ ozs.	52	1	20
Sourdough rye, Arnold's, 1 slice, 1½ ozs.	57	1	21
White, 1 slice, 1 oz.	70 (av)	1	12
100% stoneground whole wheat, 1 slice, 1½ ozs.	53	1	15
Whole wheat, 1 slice, 1 oz.	69 (av)	1	13
Bread stuffing from mix, 2 ozs.	74	5	13
Breakfast cereals			
All-Bran with extra fiber™, Kellogg's, ½ cup, 1 oz.	51	1	20
Bran Buds with Psyllium™, Kellogg's, ½ cup, 1 oz.	45	1	24
Bran Flakes, Post, ⅔ cup, 1 oz.	74	1	22
Cheerios™, General Mills, 1 cup, 1 oz.	74	2	23
Cocoa Krispies™, Kellogg's, 1 cup, 1 oz.	77	1	27
Corn Bran™, Quaker Crunchy, ¾ cup, 1 oz.	75	1	23
Corn Chex™, Nabisco, 1 cup, 1 oz.	83	0	26
Corn Flakes™, Kellogg's, 1 cup, 1 oz.	84 (av)	0	24
Cream of Wheat, instant, 1 packet, 1 oz.	74	0	21

FOOD	GLYCEMIC INDEX	FAT (G PER SVG.)	CHO (G PER SVG.)
Cream of Wheat, old fashioned, ¾ cup, cooked, 6 ozs.	66	0	21
Crispix™, Kellogg's, 1 cup, 1 oz.	87	0	25
Frosted Flakes™, Kellogg's, ¾ cup, 1 oz.	55	0	28
Golden Grahams™, General Mills, ¾ cup, 1.6 ozs.	71	1	25
Grapenuts™, Post, ¼ cup, 1 oz.	67	1	27
Grapenuts Flakes™, Post, ¾ cup, 1 oz.	80	1	24
Life™, Quaker, ¾ cup, 1 oz.	66	1	25
Muesli, natural muesli, ⅔ cup, 1½ ozs.	56	3	28
Muesli, toasted, ⅔ cup, 2 ozs.	43	10	41
Multi-Bran Chex™, General Mills, 1 cup, 2.1 ozs.	58	1.5	49
Oat bran, raw, 1 tablespoon	55	1	7
Oat bran™, Quaker Oats, ¾ cup, 1 oz.	50	1	23
Oatmeal (made with water), old fashioned, cooked, ½ cup, 4 ozs.	49 (av)	1	12
Oats, 1-minute, Quaker Oats, 1 cup, cooked	66	2	25
Puffed Wheat™, Quaker, 2 cups, 1 oz.	67	0	22
Raisin Bran™, Kellogg's, ¾ cup, 1 oz.	73	0	32
Rice bran, 1 tablespoon	19	2	5
Rice Chex™, General Mills, 1¼ cups, 1 oz.	89	0	27
Rice Krispies™, Kellogg's, 1¼ cups, 1 oz.	82	0	26
Shredded wheat, spoonsize, ⅔ cup, 1.2 ozs.	58	0	27
Shredded Wheat™, Post, 1 oz.	83	1	23
Smacks™, Kellogg's, ¾ cup, 1 oz.	56	1	24
Special K™, Kellogg's, 1 cup, 1 oz.	66	0	22
Team Flakes™, Nabisco, ¾ cup, 1 oz.	82	0	25
Total™, General Mills, ¾ cup, 1 oz.	76	1	24
Weetabix™, 2 biscuits, 1.2 ozs.	75	1	28
Buckwheat groats, cooked, ½ cup, 2.7 ozs.	54 (av)	1	20
Bulgur, cooked, ⅔ cup, 4 ozs.	48 (av)	0	23
Bun, hamburger, 1 prepacked bun, 1.7 ozs.	61	2	22
Butter beans, boiled, ½ cup, 4 ozs.	31 (av)	0	16
Cakes			
Angel food cake, 1 slice, 1/12 cake, 1 oz.	67	trace	17
Banana bread, 1 slice, 3 ozs.	47	7	46
Pound cake, homemade, 1 slice, 3 ozs.	54	15	42
Sponge cake, 1 slice, 1/12 cake, 2 ozs.	46	4	32
Capellini pasta, cooked, 1 cup, 6 ozs.	45	1	53
Cantaloupe, raw, ¼ small, 6½ ozs.	65	0	16

Food	Glycemic Index	Fat (g per svg.)	CHO (g per svg.)
Carrots, peeled, boiled, canned, ½ cup, 2.4 ozs.	49	0	3
Carrots, peeled, boiled, canned, ½ cup, 2.4 ozs.	49	0	3
Cereal grains			
Barley, pearled, boiled, ½ cup, 2.6 ozs.	25 (av)	0	22
Bulgur, cooked, ½ cup, 3 ozs.	48 (av)	0	17
Couscous, cooked, ½ cup, 3 ozs.	65 (av)	0	21
Corn			
Cornmeal, whole grain, from mix, cooked, ⅓ cup, 1.4 ozs.	68	1	30
Sweet corn, canned, drained, ½ cup, 3 ozs.	55 (av)	1	15
Taco shells, 2 shells, 1 oz.	68	5	17
Rice			
Basmati, white, boiled, 1 cup, 6 ozs.	58	0	50
Brown, 1 cup, 6 ozs.	55 (av)	0	37
Converted™, Uncle Ben's, 1 cup, 6 ozs.	44	0	38
Instant, cooked, 1 cup, 6 ozs.	87	0	37
Long grain, white, 1 cup, 6 ozs.	56 (av)	0	42
Parboiled, 1 cup, 6 ozs.	48	0	38
Rice cakes, plain, 3 cakes, 1 oz.	82	1	23
Short grain, white, 1 cup, 6 ozs.	72	0	42
Chana dal, ½ cup, 4 ozs.	8	3	28
Cheerios™, General Mills, breakfast cereal, 1 cup, 1 oz.	74	2	23
Cherries, 10 large cherries, 3 ozs.	22	0	10
Chickpeas (garbanzo beans),canned, drained, ½ cup, 4 ozs.	42	2	15
boiled, ½ cup, 3 ozs.	33 (av)	2	23
Chocolate butterscotch muffin, low fat from mix, 1 muffin	53	4	29
Chocolate, bar, 1½ ozs.	49	14	26
Chocolate Flavor, Nestle Quik™ (made with water), 3 teaspoons	53	0	14
Coca-Cola™, soft drink, 1 can	63	0	39
Cocoa Krispies™, Kellogg's, breakfast cereal, 1 cup, 1 oz.	77	1	27
Corn			
Cornmeal, cooked from mix, ⅓ cup, 1.4 ozs.	68	1	30
Sweet corn, canned and drained, ½ cup, 3 ozs.	55 (av)	1	15
Corn Bran™, Quaker Crunchy, breakfast cereal, ¾ cup, 1 oz.	75	1	23
Corn Chex™, General Mills, breakfast cereal, 1 cup, 1 oz.	83	0	26
Corn chips, 1 oz.	72	10	16
Corn Flakes™, Kellogg's, breakfast cereal, 1 cup, 1 oz.	84 (av)	0	24
Cornmeal, from mix, cooked, ⅓ cup, 1.4 ozs.	68	1	30

Food	Glycemic Index	Fat (g per svg.)	CHO (g per svg.)
Cookies			
Graham crackers, 4 squares, 1 oz.	74	3	22
Milk Arrowroot, 3 cookies, ½ oz.	69	2	9
Oatmeal, 1 cookie, ⅔ oz.	55	3	12
Shortbread, 4 small cookies, 1 oz.	64	7	19
Social Tea™ biscuits, Nabisco, 4 cookies, ⅔ oz.	55	3	13
Vanilla wafers, 7 cookies, 1 oz.	77	4	21
see also Crackers			
Couscous, cooked, ⅔ cup, 4 ozs.	65 (av)	0	21
Crackers			
Crispbread, 3 crackers, ⅔ oz.	81	0	15
Kavli™ All Natural Whole Grain Crispbread, 4 wafers, 1 oz.	71	1	16
Premium soda crackers, saltine, 8 crackers, 1 oz.	74	3	17
Rice cakes, plain, 3 cakes, 1 oz.	82	1	23
Ryvita™ Tasty Dark Rye Whole Grain Crisp Bread, 2 slices, ⅔ oz.	69	1	16
Stoned wheat thins, 3 crackers, ⅕ oz.	67	2	15
Water cracker, Carr's, 3 king size crackers, ⅗ oz.	78	2	18
Cream of Wheat, instant, 1 packet, 1 oz.	74	0	21
Cream of Wheat, old fashioned, ¾ cup, cooked, 6 ozs.	66	0	21
Crispix™, Kellogg's, breakfast cereal, 1 cup, 1 oz.	87	0	25
Croissant, medium, 1.2 ozs.	67	14	27
Custard, ½ cup, 4.4 ozs.	43	4	24
Dairy foods and nondairy substitutes			
Ice cream, 10% fat, vanilla, ½ cup, 2.2 ozs.	61 (av)	7	16
Ice milk, vanilla, ½ cup, 2.2 ozs.	50	3	15
Milk, whole, 1 cup, 8 ozs.	27 (av)	9	11
skim, 1 cup, 8 ozs.	32	0	12
chocolate flavored, 1%, 1 cup, 8 ozs.	34	3	26
Pudding, ½ cup, 4.4 ozs.	43	4	24
Soy milk, 1 cup, 8 ozs.	31	7	14
Tofu frozen dessert (nondairy), low fat, ½ cup, 2 ozs.	115	1	21
Yogurt			
nonfat, fruit flavored, with sugar, 8 ozs.	33	0	30
nonfat, plain, artificial sweetener, 8 ozs.	14	0	17
nonfat, fruit flavored, artificial sweetener, 8 ozs.	14	0	16
Dates, dried, 5, 1.4 ozs.	103	0	27
Doughnut with cinnamon and sugar, 1.6 ozs.	76	11	29
Fanta™, soft drink, 1 can	68	0	47

Food	Glycemic Index	Fat (g per svg.)	CHO (g per svg.)
Fava beans, frozen, boiled, ½ cup, 3 ozs.	79	0	17
Fettucine, cooked, 1 cup, 6 ozs.	32	1	57
Fish sticks, frozen, oven-cooked, fingers, 3½ ozs.	38	14	24
Flan cake, ½ cup, 4 ozs.	65	5	23
French baguette bread, 1 oz.	95	0	15
French fries, large, 4.3 ozs.	75	22	46
Frosted Flakes™, Kellogg's, breakfast cereal, ¾ cup, 1 oz.	55	0	28
Fructose, pure, 3 packets	23 (av)	0	10
Fruit cocktail, canned in natural juice, ½ cup, 4 ozs.	55	0	15
Fruits and fruit products			
Agave nectar (90% fructose syrup), 1 tablespoon	11	0	16
Apple, 1 medium, 5 ozs.	38 (av)	0	18
Apple, dried, 1 oz.	29	0	24
Apple juice, unsweetened, 1 cup, 8 ozs.	40	0	29
Apricots, fresh, 3 medium, 3.3 ozs.	57	0	12
canned, light syrup, 3 halves	64	0	19
dried, 1 oz.	31	0	13
Apricot jam, no added sugar, 1 tablespoon	55	0	17
Banana, raw, 1 medium, 5 ozs.	55 (av)	0	32
Cantaloupe, raw, ¼ small, 6½ ozs.	65	0	16
Cherries, 10 large, 3 ozs.	22	0	10
Dates, dried, 5, 1.4 ozs.	103	0	27
Fruit cocktail, canned in natural juice, ½ cup, 4 ozs.	55	0	15
Grapefruit, raw, ½ medium, 3.3 ozs.	25	0	5
Grapefruit juice, unsweetened, 1 cup, 8 ozs.	48	0	22
Grapes, green, 1 cup, 3 ozs.	46 (av)	0	15
Kiwi, 1 medium, raw, peeled, 2½ ozs.	52 (av)	0	8
Mango, 1 small, 5 ozs.	55 (av)	0	19
Marmalade, 1 tablespoon	48	0	17
Orange, navel, 1 medium, 4 ozs.	44 (av)	0	10
Orange juice, 1 cup, 8 ozs.	46	0	26
Papaya, ½ medium, 5 ozs.	58 (av)	0	14
Peach, fresh, 1 medium, 3 ozs.	28	0	7
canned, natural juice, ½ cup, 4 ozs.	30	0	14
canned, light syrup, ½ cup, 4 ozs.	52	0	18
canned, heavy syrup, ½ cup, 4 ozs.	58	0	26
Pear, fresh, 1 medium, 5 ozs.	38 (av)	0	21
canned in pear juice, ½ cup, 4 ozs.	44	0	13

Food	Glycemic Index	Fat (G per svg.)	CHO (G per svg.)
Pineapple, fresh, 2 slices, 4 ozs.	66	0	10
Pineapple juice, unsweetened, canned, 8 ozs.	46	0	34
Plums, 1 medium, 2 ozs.	39 (av)	0	7
Raisins, ¼ cup, 1 oz.	64	0	28
Strawberry jam, 1 tablespoon	51	0	18
Watermelon, 1 cup, 5 ozs.	72	0	8
Gatorade™ sports drink, 1 cup, 8 ozs.	78	0	14
Glucose powder, 2½ tablets	102	0	10
Gluten-free bread, 1 slice, 1 oz.	90	1	18
Golden Grahams™, General Mills, ¾ cup, 1.6 ozs.	71	1	25
Granola Bars™, Quaker Chewy, 1 oz.	61	2	23
Gnocchi, cooked, 1 cup, 5 ozs.	68	3	71
Graham crackers, 4 squares, 1 oz.	74	3	22
Grapefruit, raw, ½ medium, 3.3 ozs.	25	0	5
Grapefruit juice unsweetened, 1 cup, 8 ozs.	48	0	22
Grapenuts™, Post, breakfast cereal, ¼ cup, 1 oz.	67	1	27
Grapenuts Flakes™, Post, breakfast cereal, ¾ cup, 1 oz.	80	1	24
Grapes, green, 1 cup, 3.3 ozs.	46 (av)	0	15
Green pea soup, canned, ready to serve, 1 cup, 9 ozs.	66	3	27
Hamburger bun, 1 prepacked bun, 1½ ozs.	61	2	22
Honey, 1 tablespoon	58	0	16
Ice cream, 10% fat, vanilla, ½ cup, 2.2 ozs.	61 (av)	7	16
Ice milk, vanilla, ½ cup, 2.2 ozs.	50	3	15
Isostar, 1 cup, 8 ozs.	73	0	18
Jelly beans, 10 large, 1 oz.	80	0	26
Kaiser rolls, 1 roll, 2 ozs.	73	2	34
Kavli™ All Natural Whole Grain Crispbread, 4 wafers, 1 oz.	71	1	16
Kidney beans, red, boiled, ½ cup, 3 ozs.	27 (av)	0	20
Kidney beans, red, canned and drained, ½ cup, 4.3 ozs.	52	0	19
Kiwi, 1 medium, raw, peeled, 2½ ozs.	52 (av)	0	8
Kudos Granola Bars™ (whole grain), 1 bar, 1 oz.	62	5	20
Lactose, pure, ⁷⁄₁₀ oz.	46 (av)	0	10
Lentil soup, Unico, canned, 1 cup, 8 ozs.	44	1	24
Lentils, green and brown, boiled, ½ cup, 3 ozs.	30 (av)	0	16
Lentils, red, boiled, 1.4 cup, 4 ozs.	26 (av)	0	27
Life™, Quaker, breakfast cereal, ¾ cup, 1 oz.	66	1	25
Life Savers™, roll candy, 6 pieces, peppermint	70	0	10
Light deli (American) rye bread, 1 slice, 1 oz.	68	1	16

Food	Glycemic Index	Fat (g per svg.)	CHO (g per svg.)
Lima beans, baby, frozen, ½ cup, 3 ozs.	32	0	17
Linguine pasta, thick, cooked, 1 cup, 6 ozs.	46 (av)	1	56
Linguine pasta, thin, cooked, 1 cup, 6 ozs.	55 (av)	1	56
M&M's Chocolate Candies Peanut™, 1.7 oz. package	33	13	30
Macaroni and Cheese Dinner™, Kraft packaged, cooked, 1 cup, 7 ozs.	64	17	48
Macaroni, cooked, 1 cup, 6 ozs.	45	1	52
Maltose (maltodextrin), pure, 2½ teaspoons	105	0	10
Mango, 1 small, 5 ozs.	55 (av)	0	19
Marmalade, 1 tablespoon	48	0	17
Mars Almond Bar™, 1.8 ozs.	65	12	31
Melba toast, 6 pieces, 1 oz.	70	2	23
Milk, whole, 1 cup, 8 ozs.	27 (av)	9	11
skim, 1 cup, 8 ozs.	32	0	12
chocolate flavored, 1%, 1 cup, 8 ozs.	34	3	26
Milk Arrowroot, 3 cookies, ½ oz.	63	2	9
Millet, cooked, ½ cup, 4 ozs.	71	1	2
Muesli, breakfast cereal, toasted, ⅔ cup, 2 ozs.	43	10	41
Muesli, non-toasted, ⅔ cup, 1½ ozs.	56	3	28
Multi-Bran Chex™, General Mills, 1 cup, 2.1 ozs.	58	1.5	49
Muffins			
Apple cinnamon, from mix, 1 muffin, 2 ozs.	44	8	33
Apricot and honey, low fat, from mix, 1 muffin	60	4	27
Banana, oat and honey, low fat, from mix, 1 muffin	65	4	27
Blueberry, 1 muffin, 2 ozs.	59	4	27
Chocolate butterscotch, low fat, from mix, 1 muffin	53	4	29
Oat and raisin, low fat, from mix, 1 muffin	54	3	28
Oat bran, 1 muffin, 2 ozs.	60	4	28
Mung beans, boiled, ½ cup, 3½ ozs.	38	1	18
Natural Ovens 100% Whole Grain bread, 1 slice, 1.2 ozs.	51	0	17
Natural Ovens Hunger Filler bread, 1 slice, 1.2 ozs.	59	0	16
Natural Ovens Natural Wheat bread, 1 slice, 1.2 ozs.	59	0	16
Natural Ovens Happiness bread, 1 slice, 1.1 ozs.	63	0	15
Navy beans, boiled, ½ cup, 3 ozs.	38 (av)	0	
Nutella™ (spread), 2 tablespoons, 1 oz.	33	9	19
Oat and raisin muffin, low fat from mix, 1 muffin	54	3	28
Oat bran, 1 tablespoon	55	1	7

Food	Glycemic Index	Fat (g per svg.)	CHO (g per svg.)
Oat bran™, Quaker Oats, breakfast cereal, ¾ cup, 1 oz.	50	1	23
Oat bran, 1 muffin, 2 ozs.	60	4	28
Oatmeal (made with water), old fashioned, cooked, 1 cup, 8 ozs.	49	2	26
Oatmeal cookie, 1, ⅔ oz.	55	3	12
Oats, 1-minute, Quaker Oats, 1 cup, cooked	66	2	25
Orange, navel, 1 medium, 4 ozs.	44 (av)	0	10
Orange syrup, diluted, 1 cup	66	0	20
Orange juice, 1 cup, 8 ozs.	46	0	26
Papaya, ½ medium, 5 ozs.	58 (av)	0	14
Parsnips, boiled, ½ cup, 2½ ozs.	97	0	15
Pasta			
Capellini, cooked, 1 cup, 6 ozs.	45	1	53
Fettucine, cooked, 1 cup, 6 ozs.	32	1	57
Gnocchi, cooked, 1 cup, 5 ozs.	68	3	71
Linguine thick, cooked, 1 cup, 6 ozs.	46 (av)	1	56
Linguine thin, cooked, 1 cup, 6 ozs.	55 (av)	1	56
Macaroni, cooked, 1 cup, 5 ozs.	45	1	52
Macaroni & Cheese Dinner™, Kraft, packaged, cooked, 1 cup, 7 ozs.	64	17	48
Ravioli, meat-filled, cooked, 1 cup, 9 ozs.	39	8	32
Spaghetti, white, cooked, 1 cup, 6 ozs.	41 (av)	1	52
Spaghetti, whole wheat, cooked, 1 cup, 6 ozs.	37 (av)	1	48
Spirali, durum, cooked, 1 cup, 6 ozs.	43	1	56
Star Pastina, cooked, 1 cup, 6 ozs.	38	1	56
Tortellini, cheese, cooked, 8 ozs.	50	6	26
Vermicelli, cooked, 1 cup, 6 ozs.	35	0	42
Pastry, flaky, ⅛ of double crust, 2 ozs.	59	15	24
Pea soup, split with ham, canned, 1 cup, Wil-Pak Foods, 5½ ozs.	66	7	56
Peach, fresh, 1 medium, 3 ozs.	28	0	7
canned, heavy syrup, ½ cup, 4 ozs.	58	0	26
canned, light syrup, ½ cup. 4 ozs.	52	0	18
canned, natural juice, ½ cup, 4 ozs.	30	0	14
Peanuts, roasted, salted, ½ cup, 2½ ozs.	14 (av)	38	16
Pear, fresh, 1 medium, 5 ozs.	38 (av)	0	21
canned in pear juice, ½ cup, 4 ozs.	44	0	13
Peas, green, fresh, frozen, boiled, ½ cup, 2.7 ozs.	48 (av)	0	11
Peas dried, boiled, ½ cup, 2 ozs.	22	0	7

Food	Glycemic Index	Fat (g per svg.)	CHO (g per svg.)
Pineapple, fresh, 2 slices, 4 ozs.	66	0	10
Pineapple juice, unsweetened, canned, 8 ozs.	46	0	34
Pinto beans, canned, ½ cup, 4 ozs.	45	1	18
Pinto beans, soaked, boiled, ½ cup, 3 ozs.	39	0	22
Pita bread, whole wheat, 6½ inch loaf, 2 ozs.	57	2	35
Pizza, cheese and tomato, 2 slices, 8 ozs.	60	22	56
Plums, 1 medium, 2 ozs.	39 (av)	0	7
Popcorn, light, microwave, 2 cups (popped)	55	3	12
Potatoes			
Desirée, peeled, boiled, 1 medium, 4 ozs.	101	0	13
French fries, large, 4.3 ozs.	75	26	49
instant mashed potatoes, Carnation Foods™, ½ cup, 3½ ozs.	86	2	14
new, unpeeled, boiled, 5 small (cocktail), 6 ozs.	62 (av)	0	23
new, canned, drained, 5 small, 6 ozs.	61	0	23
red-skinned, peeled, boiled, 1 medium, 4 ozs.	88 (av)	0	15
red-skinned, baked in oven (no fat), 1 medium, 4 ozs.	93 (av)	0	15
red-skinned, mashed, ½ cup, 4 ozs.	91 (av)	0	16
red-skinned, microwaved, 1 medium, 4 ozs.	79	0	15
sweet potato, peeled, boiled, ½ cup mashed, 3 ozs.	54 (av)	0	20
white-skinned, peeled, boiled, 1 medium, 4 ozs.	63 (av)	0	24
white-skinned, with skin, baked in oven (no fat), 1 medium, 4 ozs.	85 (av)	0	30
white-skinned, mashed, ½ cup, 4 ozs.	70 (av)	0	20
white-skinned, with skin, microwaved, 1 medium, 4 ozs.	82	0	29
Sebago, peeled, boiled, 1 medium, 4 ozs.	87	0	13
Potato chips, plain, 14 pieces, 1 oz.	54 (av)	11	15
Pound cake, 1 slice, homemade, 3 ozs.	54	15	42
Power Bar™, Performance, Chocolate, 1 bar	58	2	45
Premium saltine crackers, 8 crackers, 1 oz.	74	3	17
Pretzels, 1 oz.	83	1	22
Puffed Wheat™, Quaker, breakfast cereal, 2 cups, 1 oz.	67	0	22
Pumpernickel bread, whole grain, 2 slices	51	2	30
Pumpkin, peeled, boiled, mashed, ½ cup, 4 ozs.	75	0	6
Raisins, ¼ cup, 1 oz.	64	0	28
Raisin Bran™, Kellogg's, breakfast cereal, ¾ cup, 1.3 ozs.	73	0	32
Ravioli, meat-filled, cooked, 1 cup, 9 ozs.	39	8	32
Rice			
Basmati, white, boiled, 1 cup, 7 ozs.	58	0	50

Food	Glycemic Index	Fat (g per svg.)	CHO (g per svg.)
Brown, 1 cup, 6 ozs.	55 (av)	0	37
Converted™, Uncle Ben's, 1 cup, 6 ozs.	44	0	38
Instant, cooked, 1 cup, 6 ozs.	87	0	37
Long grain, white, 1 cup, 6 ozs.	56 (av)	0	42
Parboiled, 1 cup, 6 ozs.	48	0	38
Rice bran, 1 tablespoon	19	2	5
Rice cakes, plain, 3 cakes, 1 oz.	82	1	23
Short grain, white, 1 cup, 6 ozs.	72	0	42
Rice Chex™, General Mills, breakfast cereal, 1¼ cups, 1 oz.	89	0	27
Rice Krispies™, Kellogg's, breakfast cereal, 1¼ cups, 1 oz.	82	0	26
Rice vermicelli, cooked, 6 ozs.	58	0	48
Roll (bread), Kaiser, 1 roll, 2 ozs.	73	2	39
Romano (cranberry) beans, boiled, ½ cup, 3 ozs.	46	0	21
Rutabaga, peeled, boiled, ½ cup, 2.6 ozs.	72	0	3
Rye bread, 1 slice, 1 oz.	65	1	15
Ryvita™ Tasty Dark Rye Whole Grain Crisp Bread, 2 slices, ⅔ oz.	69	1	16
Sausages, smoked link, pork and beef, fried, 2½ ozs.	28	29	5
Semolina, cooked, ⅔ cup, 6 ozs.	55	0	17
Shortbread, 4 small cookies, 1 oz.	64	7	19
Shredded Wheat™, Post, breakfast cereal, 1 oz.	83	1	23
Shredded wheat, 1 biscuit, ⅚ oz.	62	0	19
Skittles Original Fruit Bite Size Candies™, 2.3 oz. pk.	70	3	59
Smacks™, Kellogg's, breakfast cereal, ¾ cup, 1 oz.	56	1	24
Snickers™, 2.2 oz. bar	41	15	36
Social Tea™ biscuits, Nabisco, 4 cookies, ⅔ oz.	55	3	13
Soft drink, Fanta™, 1 can, 12 oz.	68	0	47
Soups			
Black bean soup, ½ cup, 4½ ozs.	64	2	19
Green pea soup, canned, ready to serve, 1 cup, 9 ozs.	66	3	27
Lentil soup, Unico, canned, 1 cup, 8 ozs.	44	1	24
Pea soup, split, with ham, Wil-Pak Foods, 1 cup, 5½ ozs.	66	7	56
Tomato soup, canned, 1 cup, 9 ozs.	38	4	33
Sourdough bread, 1 slice, 1½ ozs.	52	1	20
Rye bread, Arnold's, 1 slice, 1½ ozs.	57	1	21
Soy beans, boiled, ½ cup, 3 ozs.	18 (av)	7	10
Soy milk, 1 cup, 8 ozs.	31	7	14
Spaghetti, white, cooked, 1 cup	41 (av)	1	52
Spaghetti, whole wheat, cooked, 1 cup, 5 ozs.	37 (av)	1	48

Food	Glycemic Index	Fat (g per svg.)	CHO (g per svg.)
Special K™, Kellogg's, breakfast cereal, 1 cup, 1 oz.	66	0	22
Spirali, durum, cooked, 1 cup, 6 ozs.	43	1	56
Split pea soup, 8 ozs.	60	4	38
Split peas, yellow, boiled, ½ cup, 3½ ozs.	32	0	21
Sponge cake plain, 1 slice, 3 ½ ozs.	46	4	32
Sports drinks			
Gatorade™ 1 cup, 8 ozs.	78	0	14
Isostar, 1 cup, 8 ozs.	73	0	18
Sportsplus, 1 cup, 8 ozs.	74	0	17
Sports bars			
Power Bar™, Performance Chocolate Bar, 1 bar	58	2	45
Stoned wheat thins, 3 crackers, ⅔ oz.	67	2	15
Strawberry Nestle Quik™ (made with water), 3 teaspoons	64	0	14
Strawberry jam, 1 tablespoon	51	0	18
Sucrose, 1 teaspoon	65 (av)	0	4
Syrup, fruit flavored, diluted, 1 cup	66	0	20
Sweet corn, canned, drained, ½ cup, 3 ozs.	55 (av)	1	16
Sweet potato, peeled, boiled, ½ cup mashed, 3 ozs.	54 (av)	0	20
Taco shells, 2 shells, 1 oz.	68	5	17
Tapioca pudding, boiled with whole milk, 1 cup, 10 ozs.	81	13	51
Taro, peeled, boiled, ½ cup, 2 ozs.	54	0	23
Team Flakes™, Nabisco, breakfast cereal, ¾ cup, 1 oz.	82	0	25
Tofu frozen dessert, nondairy, low fat, 2 ozs.	115	1	21
Tomato soup, canned, 1 cup, 9 ozs.	38	4	33
Tortellini, cheese, cooked, 8 ozs.	50	6	26
Total™, General Mills, breakfast cereal, ¾ cup, 1 oz.	76	1	24
Twix Chocolate Caramel Cookie™, 2, 2 ozs.	44	14	37
Vanilla wafers, 7 cookies, 1 oz.	77	4	21
Vermicelli, cooked, 1 cup, 6 ozs.	35	0	42
Vitasoy™ Soy milk, creamy original, 1 cup, 8 ozs.	31	7	14
Waffles, plain, frozen, 4 inch square, 1 oz.	76	3	13
Water crackers, 3 king size crackers, ⅔ oz.	78	2	18
Watermelon, 1 cup, 5 ozs.	72	0	8
Weetabix™ breakfast cereal, 2 biscuits, 1.2 ozs.	75	1	28
White bread, 1 slice, 1 oz.	70 (av)	1	12
Whole wheat bread, 1 slice, 1 oz.	69 (av)	1	13
Yam, boiled, 3 ozs.	51	0	31

Food	Glycemic Index	Fat (g per svg.)	CHO (g per svg.)
Yogurt			
nonfat, fruit flavored, with sugar, 8 ozs.	33	0	30
nonfat, plain, artificial sweetener, 8 ozs.	14	0	17
nonfat, fruit flavored, artificial sweetener, 8 ozs.	14	0	16

GLYCEMIC INDEX TESTING

If you are a food manufacturer, you may be interested in having the glycemic index of some of your products tested on a fee-for-service basis. For more information, contact either:

Glycaemic Index Testing Inc.
135 Mavety Street
Toronto, Ontario
Canada M6P 2L8
E-mail: thomas.wolever@utoronto.ca

or

Sydney University Glycaemic Index Research Service (SUGIRS)
Department of Biochemistry
University of Sydney
NSW 2006 Australia
Fax: (61) (2) 9351-6022
E-mail: j.brandmiller@staff.usyd.edu.au

FOR MORE INFORMATION

REGISTERED DIETITIANS

Registered Dietitians (R.D.s) are nutrition experts who provide nutritional assessment and guidance and support with weight loss. Check for the initials "R.D." after the name to identify qualified dietitians who provide the highest standard of care to their clients. The glycemic index is part of their training so all dietitians should be able to help in applying the principles in this guide, but some dietitians do specialize in certain areas. If you want more detailed advice on the glycemic index just ask the dietitian whether this is a specialty when you make your appointment.

Dietitians work in hospitals and often run their own private practices as well. For a list of dietitians in your area, contact the American Dietetic Association (ADA) Consumer Nutrition Hotline (1-800-366-1655) or visit ADA's home page at the address below. You can also check the Yellow Pages under "Dietitians."

The American Dietetic Association
216 West Jackson Boulevard
Chicago, IL 60606
Phone: 1-800-877-1600

Fax: 1-312-899-1979
Web site: http://www.eatright.org/

PRIMARY CARE PHYSICIANS

If you think you need help with a weight problem, it's always a good idea to see your primary care physician for an evaluation.

COMMUNITY SUPPORT GROUPS

Many communities offer support groups targeting people who are trying to lose weight. Your primary care physician or local hospital may be able to direct you to a support group best suited to your needs.

DIABETES ORGANIZATIONS

Extra weight can often make a diabetic condition worse. For more information about living with and controlling your diabetes, contact the following:

The American Diabetes Association
1660 Duke Street
Alexandria, VA 22314
Phone: 1-800-ADA-DISC (1-800-232-3472)
Web site: http://www.diabetes.org/

Canadian Diabetes Association
National Office
15 Toronto St. Ste. #800
Toronto, ON M5C 2E3
Phone: 1-416-363-3373
1-800-BANTING (1-800-226-8464)
Web site: http://www.diabetes.ca/

NATURAL OVENS ORDERING INFORMATION

Natural Ovens of Manitowoc
4300 County Trunk CR
P.O. Box 730
Manitowoc, WI 54221-073
Telephone: 1-800-772-0730
Fax: 920-758-2594
Web site: http://www.naturalovens.com/

ACKNOWLEDGMENTS

We would like to acknowledge the extraordinary efforts of Johanna Burani and Linda Rao, who adapted this book—and the other books in *The Glucose Revolution Pocket Guide* series—for North American readers. Together they have worked to ensure that every piece of information is accurate and appropriate for readers in the U.S. and Canada.

ABOUT THE AUTHORS

Kaye Foster-Powell, B.Sc., M. Nutr. & Diet., is an accredited dietitian-nutritionist in both public and private practice in New South Wales, Australia. A graduate of the University of Sydney (B.Sc., 1987; Masters of Nutrition and Dietetics, 1994), she has extensive experience in diabetes management and has researched practical applications of the glycemic index over the last five years. A co-author of *The Glucose Revolution* and all the titles in *The Glucose Revolution Pocket Guide* Series, she lives in Sydney, Australia.

Jennie Brand-Miller, Ph.D., Associate Professor of Human Nutrition in the Human Nutrition Unit, Department of Biochemistry, University of Sydney, Australia, is widely recognized as one of the world's leading authorities on the glycemic index. She received her B.Sc. (1975) and Ph.D. (1979) degrees from the Department of Food Science and Technology at the University of New South Wales, Australia. She is the editor of the *Proceedings of the Nutrition Society of Australia* and a member of the Scientific Consultative Committee of the Australian Nutrition Foundation. She has written more than 200 research papers, including 60 on the glycemic index of foods. A co-author of *The Glucose Revolution* and all the titles in *The Glucose*

Revolution Pocket Guide Series, she lives in Sydney, Australia.

Thomas M.S. Wolever, M.D., Ph.D., another of the world's leading researchers of the glycemic index, is Professor in the Department of Nutritional Sciences, University of Toronto, and a member of the Division of Endocrinology and Metabolism, St. Michael's Hospital, Toronto. He is a graduate of Oxford University (B.A., M.A., M.B., B.Ch., M.Sc., and D.M.) in the United Kingdom. He received his Ph.D. at the University of Toronto. His research since 1980 has focused on the glycemic index of foods and the prevention of type 2 diabetes. A co-author of *The Glucose Revolution* and all the titles in *The Glucose Revolution Pocket Guide* Series, he lives in Toronto, Canada.

Stephen Colagiuri, M.D., is the President of the Australian Diabetes Society, Director of the Diabetes Center, and head of the Department of Endocrinology, Metabolism, and Diabetes at the Prince of Wales Hospital, Randwick, New South Wales, Australia. He is a graduate of the University of Sydney (M.B.B.S., 1970) and a member of the Royal Australasian College of Physicians (1977). He has joint academic appointments at the University of New South Wales. He has authored more than 100 scientific papers, many concerned with the importance of carbohydrate in the diet of people with diabetes. A co-author of *The Glucose Revolution* and several other titles in *The Glucose Revolution Pocket Guide* Series, he lives in Sydney, Australia.

Johanna Burani, M.S., R.D., C.D.E., is a registered dietitian and certified diabetes educator with more than 10 years experience in nutritional counseling. She specializes in designing individual meal plans based on low glycemic-index food choices. The adapter of *The Glucose Revolution* and co-adapter, with Linda Rao, of all the titles in *The Glucose Revolution Pocket Guide* Series, she is the author of seven books and professional manuals, and lives in Mendham, New Jersey.

Linda Rao, M.Ed., a freelance writer and editor, has been writing and researching health topics for the past 11 years. Her work has appeared in several national publications, including *Prevention* and *USA Today*. She serves as a contributing editor for *Prevention* Magazine and is the co-adapter, with Johanna Burani, of all the titles in *The Glucose Revolution Pocket Guide* Series. She lives in Allentown, Pennsylvania.

The Glucose Revolution **begins here . . .**

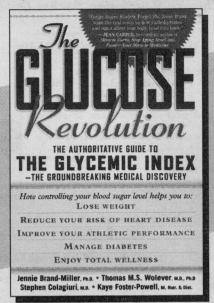

THE GLUCOSE REVOLUTION
THE AUTHORITATIVE GUIDE TO THE GLYCEMIC INDEX—
THE GROUNDBREAKING MEDICAL DISCOVERY

NATIONAL BESTSELLER!

"Forget *Sugar Busters*. Forget *The Zone*. If you want the real scoop on how carbohydrates and sugar affect your body, read this book by the world's leading researchers on the subject. It's the authoritative, last word on choosing foods to control your blood sugar."

—JEAN CARPER, best-selling author of *Miracle Brain, Miracle Cures, Stop Aging Now!* and *Food—Your Miracle Medicine*

ISBN 1-56924-660-2 • $14.95

. . . and continues with these other
Glucose Revolution Pocket Guides

The Glucose Revolution Pocket Guide to
THE TOP 100 LOW GLYCEMIC FOODS

The best of the best in low glycemic index foods
The slow digestion and gradual rise and fall in blood
sugar levels after a food with a low glycemic index has
benefits for many people. Today we know the glycemic
index of hundreds of different generic and name-brand
foods, which have been tested following a standardized
method. Now *The Top 100 Low Glycemic Foods* makes it
easy to enjoy those slowly digested carbohydrates every
day for better blood sugar control, weight loss, a healthy
heart, and peak athletic performance.
ISBN 1-56924-678-5 • $4.95

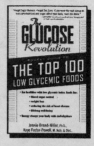

The Glucose Revolution Pocket Guide to
LOSING WEIGHT

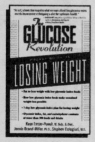

Eat yourself slim with low glycemic index foods
Not all foods are created equal when it comes to losing weight. The latest medical research shows that carbohydrates with a low glycemic index have special
advantages because they fill you up and keep you satisfied longer. This pocket guide will help you eat yourself slim with low glycemic index foods and show you
how low glycemic index foods make sustained weight
loss possible. This guide also includes a 7-day low
glycemic weight loss plan for losing weight, G.I. success stories, and the glycemic index and fat and carbohydrate
content of more than 300 foods and drinks.
ISBN 1-56924-677-7 • $4.95

The Glucose Revolution Pocket Guide to
SPORTS NUTRITION

Eat to compete better than ever before
Serious athletes and weekend warriors can gain a winning edge by manipulating the glycemic index of their
diets. Now this at-a-glance guide shows how to use the
glycemic index to boost athletic performance, enhance
stamina, and prevent fatigue. Subjects covered include
energy charging with carbohydrates, eating for com-
peting, refueling hints, menu plans and case studies,
and the glycemic index, fat and carbohydrate content
of more than 300 foods and drinks.
ISBN 1-56924-676-9 • $4.95

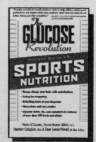

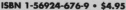